THE Q-SORT METHOD IN PERSONALITY
ASSESSMENT AND PSYCHIATRIC RESEARCH

REPRINT EDITION

Originally published by
Charles C. Thomas · Publisher
as a monograph in
The Bannerstone Division of
American Lectures in Psychology
Edited by
Molly Harrower, Ph.D.

the Q-Sort Method
in Personality Assessment
and Psychiatric Research

By

JACK BLOCK, Ph.D.

Department of Psychology
University of California
Berkeley, California

CONSULTING PSYCHOLOGISTS PRESS, INC.

577 College Avenue, Palo Alto, California 94306

Printed in the United States of America

A philosopher must be very honest to avail himself of no aid from poetry or rhetoric.

—Schopenhauer

ACKNOWLEDGMENTS

THE reader of this monograph will recognize, rather soon and then repeatedly, that its contents have been influenced in fundamental ways by the work of William Stephenson, the splendid protagonist of Q-technique. This is an inevitable indebtedness for all matters of Q-methodology have been touched by Stephenson's writings. I would like to respectfully acknowledge here the decisive impact Stephenson has had upon my own thinking.

Any work, and this one perhaps more than most, has untraceable links to colleagues and to friends. In various places in the text, I have tried to record my gratitude to individuals who have helped this effort along its way. Because so many persons have been involved at one time or another, I doubtless have failed to remember a number of names which properly should have been included. For this I am sorry.

I have better memory for the help I have received most recently. An earlier version of the present manuscript was read critically by a number of people and the present revision is, I believe, much the better for having run this friendly gauntlet. Various elliptical, tangential, and circular arguments have been excised or brought closer to earth and I have been enabled to correct certain errors before the embarrassment of seeing them in print. I have not accepted all of the suggestions these readers have offered for on certain partisan issues, I have chosen to express my own standpoint. I have been made aware, however, and I trust the manuscript now reflects this recognition, of the diversity of viewpoints that may be justified in regard to the issues treated here. Of course, for such errors as still remain, I alone am responsible. For their incisive and yet not ego-wounding help, I am much indebted to Jeanne H. Block, Lee J. Cronbach, Harrison G. Gough, Robert E. Harris, Robert R. Holt, Jean Walker Macfarlane, Norman Livson and Paul H. Mussen.

This work was supported in part by research grant M-1078 from The National Institute of Mental Health, of the National Institutes of Health, Public Health Service. The aid afforded by this grant along with the congenial surroundings of the Institute of Personality Assessment and Research under its director, Donald W. MacKinnon, helped immensely in seeing this book through. I should like, too, to record my debt to Anne Lipow and to Charlotte Mendez who have made fit for a reader a manuscript messy and patched beyond belief.

In her other, non-professional role, I am grateful, deeply, to my wife, Jeanne, for her faith and her encouragement during this enterprise. She defended me from the children for the hours I required and supported me during my vacuums of unproductivity.

JACK BLOCK

CONTENTS

THE Q-SORT METHOD IN PERSONALITY
ASSESSMENT AND PSYCHIATRIC RESEARCH

Chapter I

AN INTRODUCTION TO THE Q-SORT METHOD
OF PERSONALITY DESCRIPTION

In this monograph a language instrument is presented which *aims* to permit the comprehensive description, in contemporary psychodynamic terms, of an individual's personality in a form suitable for quantitative comparison and analysis. The language instrument consists simply of a set of personality variables—the California Q-set—together with instructions for ordering these variables so as to describe a designated person. The procedure proposed is a specific application of the rather general scaling technique due to Stephenson and known as the Q-sort method (Stephenson, 1953).

A device with the desired properties, once achieved, should have wide applicability in both research and teaching settings. In the last half-generation or so, there has been increased emphasis on an understanding of personality functioning and a disappointment in the rate of increase of knowledge in this area. Most disconcertingly, people are asking what, if anything, we know or can agree to in this field. Is there a typical mother of schizophrenics, for example? In all the talk about the "creative personality" or the "authoritarian personality," just what have people meant by these terms? What do psychiatrists and clinical psychologists intend by the notion of "ego strength"? What *really* is "hysteria"? A person dominated by a strong "need achievement" has what kind of qualities?

A short journey to the literature will indicate quickly and emphatically that questions such as these are properly to be asked if the haze of ambiguity is to be lifted. Effective communication among scientific peers is no guarantee of advance in the science but it remains a pre-condition. This premise for progress very frequently fails to obtain.

The primary virtue of the presently offered technique is that it provides a convenient means of objectifying the impressions and personality formulations of observers. By so doing, of course, the extent of agreement among people in the way in which concepts are employed can be assessed. The more important consequence, however, of this means of encoding personality evaluations is that a most rich but most complicated informational resource can come into versatile and fruitful research use in psychiatry and psychology.

Currently, personality evaluations by professionally-trained observers are in disrepute as unreliable, invalid expressions of capriciously held notions of personality. There are a number of reasons, some of them valid, why this critical attitude so dominates the psychological scene. A fundamental purpose of the present monograph is to speak out *for* the usefulness and even the inevitability of observer-evaluations as a research method. Criticisms of observer-evaluations are discussed and some ways of meeting these concerns are proposed. By way of support for our point of view, a variety of research applications of the method and principles here advocated are described.

CAUTIONARY REMARKS

It is important that the reader recognize quite clearly the special intention of the language technique—the CQ-procedure —we shall be describing. We are concerned with a method for portraying in a comprehensive and articulated fashion the personality evaluation a *professionally-trained, competent observer* forms of a subject or patient. This formulation is expressed by means of a carefully devised standard language in order to assure the possibility of comparison from observer to observer.

The variables of personality of which the standard language is composed come from no one theoretical conceptualization. The sad, existential truth of our situation is that no systematic, exhaustive and fully acceptable theory of personality exists; there is no even semi-formal system of behavior which includes the complete array of personality attributes psychologists have come to believe it is important to consider. If it did, the necessary and sufficient set of variables to portray personality functioning would be known and no problem of choice would arise. In our imperfect situation, however, some reasonable criterion for constituting an inelastic vocabulary had to be found. The solution adopted attempts, as we shall see later, to respect current informed opinions as to what aspects of personality functioning have consequence. The result is that the language developed has links to a variety of theoretical orientations; it enjoys many of the insights (but also many of the deficiencies) of contemporary clinical views and in content is reasonably familiar to workers in personality, clinical psychology and psychiatry.

The orientation of the presently proposed descriptive language is, as Lewin would say (1943), a "contemporaneous" one. *The subject is described as he appears and is understood by the observer at the time of observation.* "Historical" matters—how the subject came to evolve the personality characteristics and dynamic tendencies he now appears to have—are not in the purview of the present language technique but must be reported by other means.[1]

It is not intended to imply that the specific technique to be described outmodes special efforts to represent the essence of a personality or provides the *only* way to systematize observer-evaluations. Observer perceptions exist or will arise that must be respected even if not encompassed by a standard language. The claim of a *good* language for personality description can be only that its inexpressables are infrequent enough so that the language is essentially serviceable. As will be seen, the process by which the CQ-language evolved insures that it expresses increasingly more of the aspects of personality its users believe to be important.

Nevertheless, because of the constraints imposed whenever a standardized method is employed, the results issued by the CQ-procedure must be recognized as conditioned by the content of the CQ-set. Circumstances inevitably will arise where the vocab-

---

[1] See Chapter VIII for a brief description of a Q-set expressly designed to record, in a standard form, the salient features of an individual's personal history.

ulary provided is considered inadequate for communicating the impression the observer wishes to report. For such situations, it will always be preferable to supplement and even displace the deficient method in order to achieve the desired end.

Other methods of codifying impressions, such as conventional rating schemes (e.g., Lorr, 1953; McReynolds, Ballachey, & Ferguson, 1952; Wittenborn, 1951) and the adjective check list approach (Gough, 1960), are well known and have repeatedly demonstrated their usefulness. For many purposes, they may still be the methods of choice. It is suggested, however, that a Q-sort approach has some special advantages for the contexts of application we shall be describing, psychiatric and assessment settings and other situations where experienced and sophisticated observers are available. Support for this view will be developed subsequently.

Besides its primary purpose of bringing forward a descriptive technique believed useful in assessment and psychiatric research, the monograph serves a methodological function as well. Although the Q-sort method has been employed in numerous studies, various of its principles and intricacies have never been discussed in the literature. In the present monograph, many of the details of the Q-sort procedure, previously uncollected and unconnected, are brought together and reviewed. By so doing, some features and capabilities of the method are made public which until now have been the knowledge and lore of relatively few psychologists.

Many of the procedural details to be presented are ordinary enough but certain of the positions adopted here are controversial still for many psychologists. Rather than glide over questions of rationale, a very deliberate effort has been made to discuss them and to justify the decisions reached. Consequently, the reader is in a position to agree or to disagree with the course taken; he is not asked to accept *fiat* or *fait accompli*. This policy, however, is attended by its own disadvantages: the reader is to be burdened at times with detail and seeming digression as the program of exposition is carried through.

As a final qualification, it should be noted that our concern is expressly with the Q-sort method as it applies to observer-evaluations whereas the method has been employed much more extensively in the past as a self-descriptive device. In the latter usage, applications of the Q-sort method often have been open to certain criticisms which do not apply when the method is used to codify observer-evaluations (see, for example, Edwards [1955] on social desirability and self Q-sorts). Although much of the present methodological discussion of Q applies to both Q-sort contexts, some of the special problems of self Q-sortings are not considered here.

THE Q-SORT METHOD DESCRIBED

It may help the reader new to the Q-sort method and its relevance for personality and psychiatric research if the essentials of the method are first described and then some applications of the procedure illustrated. The later burden of understanding the rationale and details of the Q-procedure can be faced with a greater sense of resolve if its nature and usefulness are first made apparent.

In the Q-sort method, the judge or evaluator is given a set of statements or items previously developed or fixed upon. Table 1 lists the 100 items included in the present version of the CQ-set. This set of statements constitutes the entire vocabulary the judge is permitted to employ. A language, however, is more than a vocabulary; it requires a grammar as well. In order to complete the requirements for comparability of descriptions, we must insure that this vocabulary is used, at least formally, in identical ways. The special features of the CQ-method stem from this latter requirement, that descriptions in the standard vocabulary be offered also in a standard grammar so that a standard language results.

TABLE 1

THE CALIFORNIA Q-SET (FORM III)

Specified 9-point distribution (N=100):

5, 8, 12, 16, 18, 16, 12, 8, 5

1. Is critical, skeptical, not easily impressed.
2. Is a genuinely dependable and responsible person.
3. Has a wide range of interests. (N.B. Superficiality or depth of interest is irrelevant here.)
4. Is a talkative individual.

5. Behaves in a giving way toward others. (N.B. Regardless of the motivation involved.)
6. Is fastidious.
7. Favors conservative values in a variety of areas.
8. Appears to have a high degree of intellectual capacity. (N.B. Whether actualized or not.) (N.B. Originality is not necessarily assumed.)
9. Is uncomfortable with uncertainty and complexities.
10. Anxiety and tension find outlet in bodily symptoms. (N.B. If placed high, implies bodily dysfunction; if placed low, implies absence of autonomic arousal.)
11. Is protective of those close to him. (N.B. Placement of this term expresses behavior ranging from over-protection through appropriate nurturance to a laissez-faire, under-protective manner.)
12. Tends to be self-defensive.
13. Is thin-skinned; sensitive to anything that can be construed as criticism or an interpersonal slight.
14. *Genuinely* submissive; accepts domination comfortably.
15. Is skilled in social techniques of imaginative play, pretending and humor.
16. Is introspective and concerned with self as an object. (N.B. Introspectiveness *per se* does not imply insight.)
17. Behaves in a sympathetic or considerate manner.
18. Initiates humor.
19. Seeks reassurance from others.
20. Has a rapid personal tempo; behaves and acts quickly.
21. Arouses nurturant feelings in others.
22. Feels a lack of personal meaning in life.
23. Extrapunitive; tends to transfer or project blame.
24. Prides self on being "objective," rational.
25. Tends toward over-control of needs and impulses; binds tensions excessively; delays gratification unnecessarily.
26. Is productive; gets things done.
27. Shows condescending behavior in relations with others. (N.B. Extreme placement toward uncharacteristic end implies simply an *absence* of condescension, not necessarily equalitarianism or inferiority.)
28. Tends to arouse liking and acceptance in people.
29. Is turned to for advice and reassurance.
30. Gives up and withdraws where possible in the face of frustration and adversity. (N.B. If placed high, implies generally defeatist; if placed low, implies *counteractive.)*
31. Regards self as physically attractive.
32. Seems to be aware of the impression he makes on others.
33. Is calm, relaxed in manner.
34. Over-reactive to minor frustrations; irritable.
35. Has warmth; has the capacity for close relationships; compassionate.
36. Is subtly negativistic; tends to undermine and obstruct or sabotage.
37. Is guileful and deceitful, manipulative, opportunistic.
38. Has hostility toward others. (N.B. Basic hostility is intended here; mode of expression is to be indicated by other items.)

39. Thinks and associates ideas in unusual ways; has unconventional thought processes.
40. Is vulnerable to real or fancied threat, generally fearful.
41. Is moralistic. (N.B. Regardless of the particular nature of the moral code.)
42. Reluctant to commit self to any definite course of action; tends to delay or avoid action.
43. Is facially and/or gesturally expressive.
44. Evaluates the motivation of others in interpreting situations. (N.B. Accuracy of evaluation is not assumed.) (N.B. again. Extreme placement in one direction implies preoccupation with motivational interpretation; at the other extreme, the item implies a psychological obtuseness, S does not consider motivational factors.)
45. Has a brittle ego-defense system; has a small reserve of integration; would be disorganized and maladaptive when under stress or trauma.
46. Engages in personal fantasy and daydreams, fictional speculations.
47. Has a readiness to feel guilt. (N.B. Regardless of whether verbalized or not.)
48. Keeps people at a distance; avoids close interpersonal relationships.
49. Is basically distrustful of people in general; questions their motivations.
50. Is unpredictable and changeable in behavior and attitudes.
51. Genuinely values intellectual and cognitive matters. (N.B. Ability or achievement are not implied here.)
52. *Behaves* in an assertive fashion. (N.B. Item 14 reflects underlying submissiveness; this refers to overt behavior.)
53. Various needs tend toward relatively direct and uncontrolled expression; unable to delay gratification.
54. Emphasizes being with others; gregarious.
55. Is self-defeating.
56. Responds to humor.
57. Is an interesting, arresting person.
58. Enjoys sensuous experiences (including touch, taste, smell, physical contact).
59. Is concerned with own body and the adequacy of its physiological functioning.
60. Has insight into own motives and behavior.
61. Creates and exploits dependency in people. (N.B. Regardless of the techniques employed, e.g., punitiveness, over-indulgence.) (N.B. At other end of scale, item implies respecting and encouraging the independence and individuality of others.)
62. Tends to be rebellious and non-conforming.
63. Judges self and others in conventional terms like "popularity," "the correct thing to do," social pressures, etc.
64. Is socially perceptive of a wide range of interpersonal cues.
65. Characteristically pushes and tries to stretch limits; sees what he can get away with.
66. Enjoys esthetic impressions; is esthetically reactive.
67. Is self-indulgent.
68. Is basically anxious.
69. Is sensitive to anything that can be construed as a demand. (N.B. No implication of the kind of subsequent response is intended here.)

70. *Behaves* in an ethically consistent manner; is consistent with own personal standards.
71. Has high aspiration level for self.
72. Concerned with own adequacy as a person, either at conscious or unconscious levels. (N.B. A clinical judgment is required here; item 74 reflects subjective satisfaction with self.)
73. Tends to perceive many different contexts in sexual terms; eroticizes situations.
74. Is subjectively unaware of self-concern; feels satisfied with self.
75. Has a clear-cut, internally consistent personality. (N.B. *Amount* of information available before sorting is not intended here.)
76. Tends to project his own feelings and motivations onto others.
77. Appears straightforward, forthright, candid in dealing with others.
78. Feels cheated and victimized by life; self-pitying.
79. Tends to ruminate and have persistent, preoccupying thoughts.
80. Interested in members of the opposite sex. (N.B. At opposite end, item implies *absence* of such interest.)
81. Is physically attractive; good-looking. (N.B. The cultural criterion is to be applied here.)
82. Has fluctuating moods.
83. Able to see to the heart of important problems.
84. Is cheerful. (N.B. Extreme placement toward uncharacteristic end of continuum implies unhappiness or depression.)
85. Emphasizes communication through action and non-verbal behavior.
86. Handles anxiety and conflicts by, in effect, refusing to recognize their presence; repressive or dissociative tendencies.
87. Interprets basically simple and clear-cut situations in complicated and particularizing ways.
88. Is personally charming.
89. Compares self to others. Is alert to real or fancied differences between self and other people.
90. Is concerned with philosophical problems; e.g., religions, values, the meaning of life, etc.
91. Is power oriented; values power in self and others.
92. Has social poise and presence; appears socially at ease.
93a. *Behaves* in a masculine style and manner.
   b. *Behaves* in a feminine style and manner. (N.B. If subject is male, 93a. applies; if subject is female, 93b. is to be evaluated.) (N.B. again. The cultural or sub-cultural conception is to be applied as a criterion.)
94. Expresses hostile feelings directly.
95. Tends to proffer advice.
96. Values own independence and autonomy.
97. Is emotionally bland; has flattened affect.
98. Is verbally fluent; can express ideas well.
99. Is self-dramatizing; histrionic.
100. Does not vary roles; relates to everyone in the same way.

In application, the items in the CQ-set are arranged by the evaluator so as to characterize the particular person being formulated. That is, the items "are put in an order of representativeness [or significance] for the individual, those most characteristic of him being given high scores, whilst those least characteristic are scored low" (Stephenson, 1936, p. 357). Conventionally, the Q-items are printed separately on cards, a convenience which permits easy arrangement and re-arrangement of the items until the desired ordering is obtained. Because of the feature of item-*sorting*, this general scaling procedure has become known as the Q-*sort* technique. The prefixing letter—Q—has no especial significance; by historical accident, the method came to be identified this way.

The Q-sort method was devised originally by Stephenson to provide, in convenient form, data suitable for his heuristic studies in Q or obverse factor analysis. The letter—Q—was simply generalized from its original meaning of an emphasis on correlating persons to include also a method which scaled data for this correlational approach. Much confusion has been generated by the intimate connection the Q-sort method has appeared to have with a special factor analysis orientation. In fact, the method stands in its own right as a valuable scaling technique, with no necessary relation to factor analysis. Mowrer (1953) has provided an extensive historical treatment of "Q-technique" to which the interested reader is referred.

The Q-sort method imposes certain technical constraints, to be discussed later, in that the evaluator must order the Q-items into a designated number of categories and (most important) with an assigned number of items placed in each category. For the present version of the CQ-set, nine categories are employed, the number of items distributed into each category being respectively, 5, 8, 12, 16, 18, 16, 12, 8, and 5. At one end of the continuum are placed the items most characteristic of the person being described or most "salient" in describing him. At the other end of the continuum are placed the items most uncharacteristic or most "salient" in a negative sense in formulating the personality description.

After the sorting, the placement of each of the items is re-

corded on a record sheet. The categories into which the statements have been placed are themselves numbered, from 9
through *1*, with 9 by our convention referring to the most characteristic end of the continuum and the number *1* to the least
characteristic end. For each item, the number of the category
in which it was placed is recorded as that item's value in the
personality description. With the data entered in this fashion,
ready for subsequent analysis, the procedure is completed. The
Q-cards are then shuffled, preparatory to another sorting.

SOME APPLICATIONS OF THE Q-SORT METHOD
OF PERSONALITY DESCRIPTION

All of the applications to be presented in this section assume
that observer-evaluations can provide important and reliable
"measures" of personality status. Historically, there has been a
basis for questioning this assumption and so in the next chapter
we take up in some detail the matter of the observer as an instrument. For the present purpose of providing illustrations, the
reader must consider observer evaluations as both reliable and
meaningful.

1. In a personality assessment program or in the course of
psychiatric treatment, a subject or patient usually is seen by
several professional observers—psychologists, psychiatrists, and
social workers. Typically, those who have observed the subject
or patient meet in a "diagnostic council" (Murray, 1938) or staff
meeting to discuss and to integrate their several assessments.
Such meetings are rewarding, for each observer's evaluations
tend to be enriched or properly qualified by additional perceptions brought to bear upon the subject of interest.

Often, however, the additional material brought into view
confuses by its abundance. A psychotherapist in reporting his
own views may find it difficult to understand or translate into his
own terms the characterization of the patient which comes from
a psychologist's interpretation of the Thematic Apperception
Test. The social worker, of still another persuasion, also experiences difficulties in penetrating the communication barriers
unwittingly set up by the overlapping disciplines, with their
different preferred vocabularies.

The problem is not only an inter-professional one. Within a generally equivalent orientation, e.g., among psychologists, the same communication confusions and obscurities may (and do!) exist. Psychologists trained at one university may well employ a different conceptual framework in describing personality than psychologists schooled at another institution. But, as often as not, the differences between schools of thought seem to be founded on accidental differences in language usage. Alternative conceptual orientations are important and their alternative consequences warrant respect. One cannot be blandly neutral, however, with regard to phrasemaking differences which are essentially fortuitous. Important equivalences in perception may go unrecognized and genuine differences in viewpoint may be hidden.

To a suitably naive observer of the observers, the communication dilemma so resulting is reminiscent of the story about the three blind men tactually encountering different portions of that unlikely beast, the elephant. Each perceived a truth but could not assimilate it to the truths discovered by others. It would seem that a transmutation of perceptions is required if we truly intend to press for understanding. How can this be done? And done fairly?

It is suggested that the orientation and Q-set to be described in this monograph can bring together, in a useful and reasonably comprehensive way, the several points of view held by different judges or observers so that points of similarity and of difference will be made explicit. Presently, when disagreement exists among clinicians, one cannot tell of what the disagreement truly consists. The *de facto* resolution of such divergencies often appears to be simply to agree to disagree. With the procedure to be advocated, communication between and within disciplines is forced to be explicit and areas of disagreement or agreement finally can be recognized. Upon the recognition of disagreement, we may expect that subsequent discussion is more likely to be fruitful, for it can then be issue-oriented. An instance of this application is described later in this chapter.

2. As another illustration of the usefulness of the Q-sort method to be presented, let us suppose that at a psychiatric

hospital or clinic, the question is asked, What are the personality differences between patients who subsequently are successful in a suicide attempt and patients who make only abortive efforts toward suicide? Or, what are the differences between patients who improve with tranquilizers and patients who do not? Or, what are the differences between patients whose illness changes for the worse with time and those who return to a kind of adequacy? Instances of highly useful contrasts can, of course, be multiplied.

For such contrasts, Q-sorts previously collected on a routine basis could provide abundant, relevant and easily analyzed information. Most important, the Q-information would be logically independent of the basis for constituting the groups to be compared. Consequently, the results obtained by the analysis of the Q-data would have substantial and unequivocal significance.

This research possibility would not be difficult to implement. The simple requirement is that each patient coming through for the conventional hospital "work-up" routinely be described by means of the Q-sort method, a chore requiring fifteen or twenty minutes per patient once the clinician formulating the description has gained some experience with the technical details of the method. The Q-description could be based upon psychological tests, on intake interviews, psychotherapy reports, life history accounts or other sources of information. In time, a most substantial amount of qualified, yet clinical judgments would accrue, to serve as a multifaceted informational resource, whenever some interesting independent basis for establishing comparison groups is noted.

This approach can be applied rather generally in assessment contexts and not simply within psychiatric settings. Thus, a study at the Institute of Personality Assessment and Research (IPAR) will permit the difference between practicing physicians judged as "superior" and physicians judged as "average" to be stated in terms of Q-descriptions formulated at the time these physicians were *applicants* to medical school. Another research has compared the Q-sort character formulations of effective and ineffective liars, as independently measured by psychophysiological means (Block, 1957c). To indicate the range of this application, other studies have been investigated, via comparison of Q-personality descriptions, the significance of rash and cautious decision-making (Block & Petersen, 1955a); conforming and non-conforming behavior (Crutchfield, 1955); the tendency to rely upon external visual fields rather than proprioceptive cues in determining the true vertical (Crutchfield, Woodworth and Albrecht, 1958); the personalities of schizophrenogenic and neurotogenic parents (Block, J. H., Patterson, Block, J., & Jackson, 1958); the difference between dentists who use hypnosis in their practice and dentists who do not (Borland & Hardyck, 1960); high and low scores on a variety of standard and experimental questionnaire scales (Block & Bailey, 1954; Block & Bailey, 1955; Block & Gough, 1955; Block & Petersen, 1955b); over-all competence in a psychiatrist and competence in a psychiatrist specifically with respect to his function as a psychotherapist (Knupfer, Jackson, & Krieger, 1959), and so on.

3. A third application of the Q-method involves contrasts of certain Q-sorts against a Q-standard separately and independently evolved. The result is a "similarity" or "distance" score which expresses in a useful fashion a relation of interest.

For example, in teaching a course on Rorschach or MMPI interpretation, the instructor must somehow come to some judgment of the appropriateness or inappropriateness of the interpretations offered by his students. This is a frustrating and time-consuming undertaking. Some students may concentrate on certain features of the test protocol while others manifest alternative emphases. Consequently, the personality interpretations issuing are not strictly comparable. Of course, there is the additional contribution to dismay made by the idiosyncratic and hence motley language habits of the interpreters. How shall psychological test interpretations then be compared?

If the instructor is willing to accept himself as a frame of reference, or can enlist a number of acknowledged experts as a standard of veridicality, the relevant comparisons are readily made by means of the Q-sort method. Each test interpretation, conveyed by means of the Q-language, is evaluated against this criterion of "truth," which is also expressed in Q-terms. The index of equivalence thus achieved is a convenient summary expression of the congruence of the compared interpretations.

This kind of application—relating an obtained Q-sort to a criterion formulated in the Q-language—is a highly versatile one. Approachable by this means are such questions as, Are mothers of schizophrenic children like the schizophrenic mother hypothesized in the psychiatric literature? (Block, J. H., Patterson, Block, J., & Jackson, 1958); Can diagnosis of psychiatric patients be done mechanically but configurationally? (Halbower, 1955; Meehl, 1956; Enright, 1959); Can subjects be evaluated retrospectively on dimensions or with reference to constructs not anticipated at the time of original data collection? (Block, 1957a); Do individuals scoring highly on an inventory measure of authoritarianism prove to have the personality structure proposed and delineated in The Authoritarian Personality?[2] Other research questions having to do with the similarity or difference of actual individuals to specified "scoring keys" can of course be generated at length.

4. Our final exemplification of a Q-application deals with the brambly problem of typology. Whether we will or not, psychologists think in typological terms, if only because of the abstractional convenience the notion of types provides. There are "bright" people and "stupid" people; "repressers" and "intellectualizers"; "introverts" and "extroverts"; "achievers" and "affiliators." Indeed, in a very genuine sense, the clinical emphasis on "the uniqueness of the individual" asserts that every person is a type unto himself.

Now, the implications of the typological point of view are not immediately obvious, as Cattell has pointed out (Cattell, 1952). The fundamental issue appears to be whether a type concept represents simply a language or communication convenience or whether it represents genuine divergencies in the psychological organization characterizing certain kinds of individuals (Block, 1955b). If "types" in this latter sense of the term exist, then this fact must be recognized and respected for the psychological laws that characterize one type of personality may be quite different

---

[2] Unpublished IPAR analyses.

from the psychological laws that characterize another type. Cronbach has expressed this point well: "nonchance relations cannot be perceived when fundamentally different organisms are shuffled together in a sample" (1953, p. 388).

In large part, the issues here can be approached empirically, to see whether a genuine typology is in fact present in a given data-matrix. For the present, we simply call attention to *the extreme convenience of Q-data for research on issues in this domain.* One can ask such questions as, Are creative individuals typologically uniform or are they as diverse in their personalities as a sample of highly intelligent but not expressly creative individuals? The studies presently underway at the University of California's Institute of Personality Assessment and Research will provide data on this and related questions. Have psychiatrists in their theorizing on parental determinants of schizophrenia come to some agreement or is there a fundamental difference among them in the views held? (Jackson, Block, J., Block, J. H., & Patterson, 1958); What are the fundamental types of patients coming to a particular out-patient clinic or to a particular psychiatric hospital? (Monro, 1955); and so on.

Having identified the homogeneous subgroups within a larger sample, it then becomes feasible to study the independent correlates of subgroup membership or the relationship among variables as a function of subgroup. For example, do individuals who as adults have rather similar personalities evolve from similar child-rearing contexts? (Dalaba, 1960); Is the relationship between inability to delay gratification on the one hand and introspectiveness and fantasy capacity on the other a function of the subsample being considered or is the relationship consistent over various subgroups.[3]

TWO ILLUSTRATIONS OF THE CQ-METHOD APPLIED

In the preceding section, some possibilites for applying the Q-sort procedure have been mentioned but still in highly general, allusive terms. Here we offer in more detail two illustrations of how the proposed standard language brings about in a useful

---

[3] Work in progress by the writer.

way the comparability of formulations we seek and provides research data otherwise unattainable.

The first illustration compares a personality formulation offered via the CQ-method with a personality formulation offered when no restriction is set upon the way the description is to be expressed. So that the reader can bring his own knowledge and perspectives into play in evaluating the relative merits and deficiencies of the two descriptions, it is convenient to use a concept rather than an actual person as a "subject." For this reason, we study the case of "the optimally adjusted person."

The second illustration compares the CQ-sort descriptions of creative women mathematicians with the CQ-descriptions of women mathematicians not deemed creative. The Q-descriptions, of course, were formulated independently of knowledge of the mathematical creativity of these professional mathematicians and so the discriminating items are of substantive as well as demonstrational interest.

The Case of "the Optimally Adjusted Person"

In quite another connection, several advanced graduate students in psychology were asked to compose 200 word essays on the nature of "the optimally adjusted personality." Following this exercise, each student again expressed a description of the optimal individual but this time by means of a sorting of the elements of the CQ-language. About 15 or 20 minutes was required for the second description, appreciably less time than was required for the essays. It is informative to contrast here a pair of these descriptions.

Student G, in writing his essay, had this to say:

"The concept of the optimally adjusted person may be thought of as an *abstraction* parallel to a statistical abstraction, such as a mean, or correlation coefficient. Alternatively, the concept of the optimally adjusted person can be considered as a *composite* analogous to the image resulting from superimposing many photo-negatives of an object photographed from different perspectives. Viewed from either of these alternatives, it is not surprising to find that no one individual corresponds perfectly with the concept.

"First of all, the optimally adjusted person may be characterized by having a heightened *tolerance for dissonance* (Festinger). Stated simply, this means that he can be comfortable in situations that others would attempt to avoid. Within himself he may sense certain unresolved conflicts and seeming inconsistencies, but he is at ease with this kind of dissonance. In fact, he is more often fascinated than perplexed by these inconsistencies both in himself and others.

"A great deal of this tolerance stems from a perception and appreciation of the relativity concept, especially the relativity of social behavior. He is a master of "role playing." Often he performs the conventional and socially expected in a "tongue-in-cheek" manner. However, he would never deliberately disturb others by flouting convention. This does not imply that the optimally adjusted person lacks a sense of commitment. On the contrary, his commitments are strongly reinforced by rational considerations.

"In his social relations with others, the optimally adjusted person selects his friends with care. He is more concerned with *quality* than *quantity.* He is generally friendly and outgoing with people but he does not strive to please everyone. He is no "back-slapper" or "glad-hander." To many, his seeming casualness is often misinterpreted as aloofness.

"*Intellectually,* the optimally adjusted person is *above average.* In his field of concentration he is more *the generalist* rather than the specialist. His interests are broad and he has contact with many aspects of experience. In fact, many of these interests may appear "off-beat" to some but to him they have value and meaning. This does not imply that he glorifies the esoteric; he merely pursues those lines of interest that are most congruent to him.

"Rather than being religious in the conventional sense of the word, the optimally adjusted person tends to be humanitarian in his outlook. Religion (either of the institutional variety or not) means doing something for others. He is not preoccupied by metaphysical dilemmas or verbal quibbles. He has a broad concern for others and continually searches for ways of realizing an inner need for compassion.

"In conclusion, it appears that the concept of the optimally adjusted person expounded here is not at variance with the related concepts of the *self-actualized individual* (Maslow), the *creative personality* (Ghiselin, Vinacke), or the *fully functioning personality* (Hayakawa). In the last analysis, all of these concepts may be synonymous for a common personality structure."

Student N, in her essay on psychological optimality, said:

"An optimally adjusted person is one who has an understanding and acceptance of self and society both with their limitations and strengths. This acceptance is not a passive submission to limitations that could be overcome but an insight that distinguishes evitable and inevitable ones. He is relatively *free of defenses* and compulsions and as such is also *free to enjoy the utilization of his energies,* which gives him a feeling of self fulfillment, enriches his environment and helps overcome avoidable limitations. He does not resort to work as a means of escape nor are his energies paralyzed leading him to inactive means of escape. He is free from inner compulsions and excessive need for outer controls. He is *not embarrassed to conform nor afraid to differ.* He *can accept criticism and appreciation and is also objective in his evaluation of others.*

"He is not free from problems because he is actively engaged in life. He recognizes problems and tries to understand them. He has developed independent skills but does not find it difficult to seek help when needed. He enjoys working alone and does not find it difficult to work with others. He can play the role of receiver and giver comfortably. He accepts his role as an individual in an interdependent society.

"When differences exist between his conception of his role (age and sex role) and that defined by society he has an understanding of the differences and their reasons and he is not afraid to differ within reasonable limits and still maintains an acceptance from society because he can communicate with them. When differences are greater he moves toward the direction of bringing changes in society. When there is lack of clear definition or a variety of ways of finding a role, he does not feel lost and shows sufficient self insight and flexibility to work out the role best suited to his abilities. There is not a big gap between his level of aspiration and his abilities. His controls are internalized providing a relatively consistent value system that is not too restrictive for spontaneity nor too loose for organization and control."

Each of the preceding brief statements represents a considered effort to characterize the concept of optimal adjustment. These formulations read well and possess an intrinsic interest. But how do they compare? The first essay emphasizes such attributes as "tolerance for dissonance," "role-playing (ability)," "a sense of commitment," breadth of interest, and "humanitarianism." The second essay describes optimal adjustment in terms of freedom "from inner compulsions and excessive need for outer controls," the ability "to accept criticism and appreciation" and "also [be] objective in evaluation of others." Do we have an equivalence in evaluations here? And how shall we know?

The ambiguity in evaluating these formulations comes from two sources. The first is the inevitable circumstance that essayists have personal styles of expression and, consequently, create a translation problem for a would-be interpreter. The second (and not less important) contribution to ambiguity comes because the essayists do not focus their perceptions upon the same set of attributes in describing their "subject." The first writer says nothing in regard to, for example, the ability to accept criticism, a quality stressed by the second writer. Conversely, one can only guess as to the second essayist's views on the place of "tolerance for dissonance" in her conception of the optimally adjusted person. Yet, intuitively, there does appear to be more than a little congruence between the two characterizations we have just quoted. Consider now how this same description problem is treated by the Q-procedure.

The 26 most salient items in Student G's formulation of the optimally adjusted person are listed in Table 2. Also to be read from this table are the 26 most salient items as evaluated by Student N. For reasons of brevity, the order of the remaining 74 items in each description is not given.

TABLE 2

CQ-Items Falling in the Highest Two and Lowest Two Categories
for Student G and Student N

Q-Category	Student G	Student N
Most Characteristic (5 items)	(3) Has a wide range of interests (35) Has warmth; has the capacity for close relationships; compassionate. (51) Genuinely values intellectual and cognitive matters. (64) Is socially perceptive of a wide range of interpersonal cues. (96) Values own independence and autonomy.	(26) Is productive; gets things done. (28) Tends to arouse liking and acceptance in people. (60) Has insight into own motives and behavior. (70) *Behaves* in an ethically consistent manner; is consistent with own personal standards. (75) Has a clear-cut, internally consistent personality.
Quite Characteristic (8 items)	(17) Behaves in a sympathetic or considerate manner. (26) Is productive; gets things done. (60) Has insight into own motives and behavior. (66) Enjoys esthetic impressions; is esthetically reactive. (70) *Behaves* in an ethically consistent manner; is consistent with own personal standards. (71) Has high aspiration level for self. (77) Appears straightforward, forthright, candid in dealings with others. (83) Able to see to the heart of important problems.	(2) Is a genuinely dependable and responsible person. (32) Seems to be aware of the impression he makes on others. (33) Is calm, relaxed in manner. (35) Has warmth; has the capacity for close relationships; compassionate. (64) Is socially perceptive of a wide range of interpersonal cues. (77) Appears straightforward, forthright, candid in dealing with others. (80) Interested in members of the opposite sex. (93) *Behaves* in a masculine (feminine) style and manner.
Quite Uncharacteristic (8 items)	(23) Extrapunitive; tends to transfer or project blame. (30) Gives up and withdraws where possible in face of frustration and adversity. (40) Is vulnerable to real or fancied threat, generally fearful. (45) Has a brittle ego-defense system; has a small reserve of integration; would be disorganized or maladaptive under stress or trauma.	(10) Anxiety and tension find outlet in bodily symptoms. (12) Tends to be self-defensive. (25) Tends toward over-control of needs and impulses; binds tensions excessively; delays gratification unnecessarily. (34) Over-reactive in minor frustrations; irritable. (42) Reluctant to commit self to any definite course of action; tends to delay or avoid action.

(49) Is basically distrustful of people; questions their motivations.
(61) Creates and exploits dependency in people.
(78) Feels cheated and victimized by life; self-pitying.
(86) Handles anxiety and conflicts by in effect refusing to recognize their presence; repressive . . . tendencies.

(45) Has a brittle ego-defense system; has a small reserve of integration; would be disorganized or maladaptive under stress or trauma.
(68) Is basically anxious.
(78) Feels cheated and victimized by life; self-pitying.

Most Uncharacteristic (5 items)

(10) Anxiety and tension find outlet in bodily symptoms.
(38) Has hostility toward others.
(47) Has a readiness to feel guilty.
(59) Is concerned with own body and the adequacy of its physiological functioning.
(73) Tends to perceive many different contexts in sexual terms; eroticizes situations.

(38) Has hostility toward others.
(40) Is vulnerable to real or fancied threat, generally fearful.
(47) Has a readiness to feel guilty.
(49) Is basically distrustful of people in general; questions their motives.
(86) Handles anxiety and conflicts by, in effect, refusing to recognize their presence; repressive or dissociative tendencies.

As can be seen from the table, both essayists have now spoken in the same terms and with respect to the same set of dimensions. It is apparent that the comparison task at this point is easy and straightforward. Various methods of comparison are available. If one seeks a summary expression of the extent of over-all agreement between two descriptions, a correlation coefficient is a useful index. In the present instance, the correlation between the Q-descriptions of the two descriptions is .77, indicating appreciable convergence in their conceptualizations of optimal adjustment.

Content-wise, both judges agree that the optimally adjusted person is warm, productive, insightful, ethically consistent, perceptive, and candid. The definition, at its negative end, excludes such attributes as hostility, anxiety, fearfulness, pervasive guilt feelings, distrust, self-pity, and the use of repressive mechanisms. These items (and others not listed in Table 2) constitute the core of agreement. There are some instructive differences though, also, between the two conceptions. Student G places more value on such attributes as intelligence, esthetic reactivity and autonomy than does Student N. Student N, on the other hand, emphasizes heterosexuality, appropriateness and a lack of projectivity more than does Student G. Other differences exist but these few perhaps can indicate the different flavors of the alternative conceptualizations.

With the essays, one could only attempt to sense the nature of the equivalence between descriptions, and any opinion as to areas or extent of agreement was open to alternative interpretations. The CQ-procedure, however, as just exemplified, permits the job of comparison to be done objectively and, it is suggested, relevantly. By requiring each judge to attend to the complete range of attributes included in the language, the dangers of differential focussing are avoided. Certainly, these Q-descriptions are not so appealing to read as descriptions expressed in the less circumscribed essay form. But where previously comparisons were not directly and unequivocally possible, the Q-procedure makes them available—a most important achievement.

There remains the question of whether this accomplishment has not been achieved at excessive cost. Perhaps the objectification of comparisons is no more than that. If by this effort at objectivity we have achieved asepsis but lost relevance, then of course we are defeated by our victory. The reader can form his own impressions as to whether, in the example above, the essays or the Q-descriptions are most informative and precise in conveying the conceptions held by the individuals involved. In the later chapters, it may be noted that this question—of the balance between the costs and the gains accruing from the Q-method—is referred to often. We have been sensitive to this issue throughout the evolvement of the California Q-set and more than a little, have shaped our procedure accordingly. The ultimate judgment on this matter, of course, must come out of the crucible of empiricism.

Creativity in Women Mathematicians as Specified by the CQ-Set

As a second way of conveying concretely the CQ-method and its capabilities, we cite some results from the ongoing creativity research at IPAR, one part of which has focussed upon creativity in women and, in particular, in women mathematicians.[4]

A highly selected sample of 40 women mathematicians was intensively assessed at IPAR by a staff of psychologists. The procedures experienced by the women were comprehensive in scope and included a variety of perceptual-cognitive and experimental procedures, a battery of standard psychological tests, and some specially designed interpersonal situations (e.g., charades, group discussions, interviews). Each member of the psychological staff, at the end of the assessment, described each woman mathematician by means of the CQ-set. The several CQ-descriptions for each subject were then averaged to provide one consensus-based description for each woman.

Independently, and by a panel of mathematicians, each of the subjects previously had been carefully rated on a continuum of mathematical creativity. It is most important to note that none of the assessing psychologists had information as to the judged mathematical creativity of the subjects nor did any of the psychologists possess the personal mathematical competence to infer the subject's probable creativity rating.

The 40 scores for each CQ-item were then correlated with the independently derived ratings of creativity. Table 3 reports the Q-items significantly related to this criterion.

TABLE 3

CQ-Items Significantly Correlated with Creativity
in Women Mathematicians

Positively Correlated:

Item 39. Thinks and associates to ideas in unusual ways; has unconventional thought processes. (.64)

Item 57. Is an interesting, arresting person. (.55)

Item 62. Tends to be rebellious and non-conforming. (.51)

Item 51. Genuinely values intellectual and cognitive matters. (.49)

Item 8. Appears to have a high degree of intellectual capacity. (.46)

Item 99. Is self-dramatizing; histrionic. (.42)

Item 82. Has fluctuating moods. (.40)

Item 1. Is critical, skeptical, not easily impressed. (.38)

Item 94. Expresses hostile feelings directly. (.36)

---

[4] The writer is privileged to report these data by the courtesy of Dr. Ravenna Helson, Project Director of this study.

Item 53. Various needs tend toward relatively direct and uncontrolled expression; unable to delay gratification. (.35)

Item 46. Engages in personal fantasy and daydreams, fictional speculations. (.34)

Item 50. Is unpredictable and changeable in behavior and attitudes. (.31)

Item 65. Characteristically pushes and tries to stretch limits; sees what he can get away with. (.30)

Negatively Correlated:

Item 63. Judges self and others in conventional terms like "popularity," "the correct thing to do," social pressures, etc. (−.62)

Item 2. Is a genuinely dependable and responsible person. (−.45)

Item 17. Behaves in a sympathetic or considerate manner. (−.43)

Item 7. Favors conservative values in a variety of areas. (−.40)

Item 41. Is moralistic. (−.40)

Item 24. Prides self on being "objective," rational. (−.37)

Item 9. Is uncomfortable with uncertainty and complexities. (−.35)

Item 11. Is protective of those close to him. (−.35)

Item 70. *Behaves* in an ethically consistent manner; is consistent with own personal standards. (−.33)

These Q-results have appreciable intrinsic interest. Of the 100 items correlated with the criterion, 22 emerge as significant discriminators beyond the .05 level. The items positively correlated with creativity appear to describe an unusual, amoral, flamboyant person who, although impulsive and direct in her expression, is also moody and introverted. The items negatively correlated with creativity portray a very different kind of woman —one tied to conventionality, to internalized moral standards and the safeguards these provide against impulse expression and the uncertainties in the world. Especially striking is the similarity of these descriptions to the CQ-descriptions previously reported by Barron (1957) in a comparison of original and unoriginal Air Force officers, where originality was defined very differently by objective test performance.

A full understanding of these and related results must await completion of the many comparisons yet required to close in on the essential nature of creativity in its general and particular aspects. The purpose of presenting these preliminary results at this time will have been served if the reader has gained some additional recognition of the convenience and fruitfulness of the CQ-method in a research setting.

Chapter II

A PERSPECTIVE ON OBSERVER-EVALUATIONS
OF PERSONALITY

The Q-procedure may be viewed as essentially a kind of rating procedure, one means of quantifying observer-evaluations. Although over the years rating procedures have been tolerated as a way of expressing judgments, they have not enjoyed the best of reputations as a form of scientific data.

The aspersions that have beeen cast at methods of quantifying observer-evaluations are several and come from rather different segments of the psychological community. Three main lines of criticism have appeared. First, it has been said that observer-evaluations are not important stuff for the science of personality. The reason presumably is that the "instrument" of observation here is a human being and a properly operational science does not (or should not) let an individual serve in this capacity. According to this view, it would be far better to measure personality by some test or inventory.

A second criticism is perhaps only an extension of the first. Even if the observer could be permitted to serve as an instrument, the problem of the reproducibility of the data so gathered would then arise. The logic of science requires reproducible, intersubjective data, data which are not dependent upon a particular individual for their collection. But is it not so that observers or judges vary significantly among themselves and hence cannot provide dependable, repeatable information?

The third kind of criticism leveled against the qualification of observations comes from quite a different source. Here the argument upholds the relevance of observer-evaluations *per se* but asserts that when the formalities of observer qualification are introduced, an injustice is done to the complexly arranged information held by the observer. Rating methods—at least the traditional rating methods—do not permit proper expression of the integrated personality formulations developed by a judge. An incisive perception may be crudely used by the arbitrary rating scheme, with a resulting loss of important information. And so from this side too comes a devaluing of efforts to quantify observer-evaluations.

Sometimes, it would appear, this attitude against quantification fails to recognize that constraints are imposed by any effort at science. Such a position is effectively anti-scientific for it makes a mystique out of mystery. Each inadequacy of science is relished and its successes discounted.

On the other hand, very much of the criticism of efforts to quantify observer-evaluations has come from workers genuinely dedicated to the scientific study of personality. From them has come, as we shall see, a more valid criticism of usual methods of quantifying observer-evaluations.

Because the present monograph represents so heavy a commitment to the use of quantified evaluations by observers, it is in order to indicate why we believe them to be important and how we propose to meet the criticisms that have been offered. To this end, the present chapter has three concerns—first, it brings forward a justification of the use of observer-evaluations; second, it calls attention to a simple, effective and not new procedure by which observer-evaluations can escape the plague of subjectivity and unreproducibility; and third, it discusses the basis for the criticism that rating procedures tend to be artificial in crucial ways and are therefore inappropriate for their intended purpose. This last point, when elaborated, sets the stage for the Q-procedure as developed in this monograph.

THE IMPORTANCE OF OBSERVER-EVALUATIONS

In the study of personality, evaluations by observers continue to be used. Why is this? One reason is that observations of personality represent a most convenient, most immediate kind of data to collect, and indeed are sometimes the only kind of data available to the investigator. Another reason is that for many purposes, where criteria—the behaviors we wish to predict—

are complex in nature and predictors are poorly developed or only poorly understood, personality evaluations have proven to be the most valid predictors we possess (e.g., Holt, 1958; Campbell & Fiske, 1959).

These justifications are valid and are perhaps sufficiently powerful support for the continued usage of observer-evaluations. But there is another quite basic reason—usually left implicit— why observer-evaluations remain so dominant a procedure in personality assessment. The reason, we would suggest, is because of the intrinsic persuasiveness or "face validity" observer-evaluations possess. The face validity of a procedure is a characteristic which may on occasion be misleading but also it is a property which in many circumstances is decisive. To understand why the compelling quality *per se* of observer-evaluations is so respected, it is necessary to remark briefly on the perpetual difficulty facing operationally oriented resarchers.

In setting up any operational psychological measure, there is the problem of assuring congruence between the objective index, as it will function, and the hypothetical variable or concept that index is designed to reflect. Ideally, the measure employed should be a suitable translation or manifestation of the concept or underlying variable the investigator is seeking to study. To the extent this ideal fails to be achieved, the resulting data possess only irrelevant or ambiguous meaning.

But how can we "know" that our measure is "in fact" a sufficient measure of the hypothetical dimension in which we are interested? The answer, briefly and unhappily, is that we cannot "know" or ever be certain. This is in the nature of things, or rather in the nature of theory and theory testing (cf. e.g., Cronbach & Meehl, 1955).

Absence of certainty however by no means requires an absence of likelihood. We begin tentatively but hope that a network of specifically sought empirical relationships will emerge that is coherent with the theoretical framework that prompted the search. If and when this eventuality develops, then, in a kind of reciprocal validation, we are supported both in our theory and in the operations we have employed to give flesh to our logical skeleton.

The foregoing is simply a re-statement of some elementary principles in the philosophy of science. Its pertinence here is to emphasize the obscurity of the situation existing at the beginning of this hypothesis-testing process, before the required "nomological net" has been established.

But how do we begin? At the initial stages of the development of measures, before a consistent, interlocking array of relationships has been found which can affirm our proposed interpretation of the measure, how can we justify our particular operations?

The second brief and unhappy answer is that in the beginning we have recourse only to persuasive argument and not to proof. The required congruence between construct and index is achieved only by suggesting that congruence out of conviction that it is "appropriate" or "fruitful" to do so.

Our regress thus turns us to the question, How shall we evaluate the appropriateness or relative fruitfulness of a proposed measure? Here the answer is that, at the outset, the basis of the conviction that a measure or index is related to an underlying dimension is nothing more than and nothing less than the highly personal ground of "reasonableness"—the ability to persuade oneself and one's scientific peers of the relevance of the operations for the construct under investigation. Initially, it is the researcher's private experience that provides the criterion or basis for hypothesizing a particular operation to be a sufficient translation or manifestation of the concept being considered. Hopefully, other knowledgeable individuals then will accept, at least tentatively, the use of the proposed operation. Only later, after much empiricism, can a "reasonable" measure take on an independent status.

Thus, it is "reasonable" to suggest heart rate variability as an index of underlying anxiety. It would be less "reasonable" to propose buttoning rate as an anxiety manifestation. Conservatism is more reasonably indexed by noting an individual's political party affiliation than it is by observing the color of the shoes he wears.

To return now to our particular context and the "face validity" of observer-evaluations, it is clear that evaluations by observers, when used as indices of personality status, appear to stand in rather direct and faithful correspondence with the observer's understanding of and beliefs about how his subject (patient, social object) is placed on the dimensions of interest. This is not to say that observers, as instruments of detection, are necessarily accurate or possess truth. The point is more that observers can deal directly with the variables chosen as fundamental. Their statements, viewed now as operational indices, are close to the dimensions or concepts hypothesized as significant.

By contrast, many certainly more objective personality measures seem distant from or only trivially related to the underlying variables of concern. This continuing contrast—as much a comment on the general status of personality measurement as it is on the convincingness of observer-evaluations—is perhaps the fundamental reason why this ancient approach is still with us and still has a function to serve.

One can find in the literature measures of weight, height, attitude toward Germans, and attitude toward Chinese all employed as facets of the concept of "impulsivity" (Twain, 1957). The construct of "anxiety" is measured by the Taylor Manifest Anxiety scale in one study (Eriksen & Davids, 1955) and by a virtually equivalent scale, *scored in a reversed direction,* in another (Eriksen & Browne, 1956). The notion of "empathy" is objectified by a test which, among other exotica, asks its takers to estimate the circulation of a number of American magazines, one of which has been defunct since the date of publication of the test (Kerr & Speroff, 1951). Admittedly, these are extreme instances and our intention is not to suggest that all "objective" ways of representing important psychological constructs involve such irrelevancies or contradictions. Rather, the implication we would draw from the susceptibility to absurdity of unthinking efforts at objectivity is that a collaborative, not competitive association between observer - evaluations and "observer - less" measures is required. Because of present limitations in the realm of objective personality measurement, a place still remains for observer-evaluations as the initial standard against which "observer-less" measures may be compared.

The dean of medical school, distressed at the burgeoning of medical selection devices all of marginal validity, once sharpened the point this way: Given the efficacy of contemporary psychological tests and experiments, in choosing a mate would one be willing to trust this perhaps irreversible selection to the objective measures presently available or would a personal interview be desirable as well?

Certainly a great convenience would result from elimination of observer-evaluations. The burden of the present argument, however, is that such elimination is not possible or rather, not wise, until the special kind of contribution now offered only by observer-evaluations is attained alternatively. For the present, rather than discard observer-evaluations, it may be more productive to see if observer-evaluations can be employed in scientifically more appropriate ways.

ACHIEVING REPRODUCIBILITY OF
OBSERVER-EVALUATIONS

If observer-evaluations are to achieve usefulness as "measurements of behavior," two related requirements must be met. The observer-evaluations must not interact with or be dependent upon the idiosyncratic qualities of the observers providing the evaluations. That is, the judgements used should not be uniquely determined by the nature of the observers who just happen to be employed. In those circumstances where the professional observer is being employed as an "instrument" and the research focus is *solely* upon the qualities of the subject, this requirement has an obvious justification.[5]

The second requirement demanded of observer-evaluations is that the dimensions of evaluation be reliably indexed; the data so gathered should be substantial rather than whimsical. It must be possible to believe in the measure as a reliable concomitant of the subject's behavior and not as due to artifact or to highly special and not reproducible circumstances. Obviously, these requirements of independence and of reliability apply to *any* kind of measure proposed for scientific use.

Historically, observer-evaluations have been criticized as defi-

---

[5] For research into the nature of the judgmental process—a very different emphasis—the personal contribution of the judge of course deserves study.

cient with respect to both of these requirements. Sometimes, it has appeared that more of the judge is being expressed in the evaluation than of the subject. The reliability of observers (expressed in terms of interjudge agreement) frequently has seemed distressingly low or when high, ascribable to naive collusion among the judges. As a result of these empirical disappointments, a reputation of infidelity has developed around observer-evaluations.

The basis, or rather, the necessity of this gloomy estimation of the capabilities of observer-evaluations may be questioned, however. The fault with observer-evaluations appears to lie, not in the intrinsic validity of the data but rather in the way the data are subsequently processed. While observer-evaluations have sometimes flagrantly failed, they have worked extraordinarily well in assessment settings when they have met the methodological requirements of independence and reliability.

There exists a most simple and, it is suggested, effective way of achieving these twin goals. The technique advocated here is the expedient of gathering *multiple but independent* observer-evaluations and then taking the consensus of these several observers. This procedure is by no means new but it has been inconsistently applied and its basis and properties are improperly understood by many. Accordingly, it has suffered from both its supporters and from its detractors. Those favoring the technique have frequently misapplied or misinterpreted their results; those opposed to the procedure have been influential but have failed to acknowledge some brutely empirical findings and the larger implications of their antagonistic position. It is useful, then, to consider why we believe this method issues forth an objective, reliable—and appropriate—expression of observer-evaluations. What is the logic underlying scores so derived? What are their properties?

First, we must note that it follows quite directly, from the stipulation that judgments be independent of the particular observer, that more than one observer must be employed.[6] If the

---

[6] This statement is not strictly true. There is one very rare and perhaps unrealizable situation wherein the judgments derived from single observers may be

accusation of subjectivity is to be voided, solitary judges cannot be used and the idea of combining judgments is therefore a required one.

Required though it may be, many clinicians feel uneasy with the idea of combining judgments and there is more than a little tendency to reject the notion. Their countering argument is that separate analyses of individual judgments would reveal valid perceptions that are lost or otherwise diluted in the pooling procedure. Often, this argument against combining judgments is advanced rhetorically, with the implication that more information is to be gained by considering each observer in his vestal uniqueness rather than by mediocratizing him and his peers by combining all into a mean mean.

This argument raises both pragmatic and philosophical issues. The pragmatic question is, What is the liklihood that individualized analyses will provide more affirmative data? The question is responded to later in this section. The philosophical concern is, given that more positive results emerge from separate analyses of judges than from the analysis of a group consensus, what does this mean and where do such findings leave us—or rather, take us? This is a point relating to the nature of science and its method. It is well to state some attitudes here for they have guided much of the presently reported work.

If, in fact rather than in speculation, one particular judge is significantly more sensitive than the consensus derived from all the judges, this finding would have to be respected and used. But, in and of itself, the phenomenon would have no meaning until investigated and its why and wherefores studied. The distinction important here (it is really a continuum) is that between *prediction* and *understanding*. The first is helpful in providing leads to, and checks of, the second. But they are not the

employed in the analysis of subject differences. If a set of observers is available and may be presumed to be a proper sample from a universe of judges, and if individual observers are randomly assigned to the subjects they are then to evaluate, then the resultant subject data when treated statistically is independent of particular observer effects. This design is impractical as a rule for it requires a large group of available judges and the opportunity of randomizing assignments (or the presumption that such randomization has occurred). In addition, it provides data of less precision than when multiple judges are employed to evaluate each subject.

same. For we can predict without understanding, and understand without being able to predict.

Ultimately, in the far reaches of knowledge, prediction and understanding merge and become indistinguishable. At the present time, their separation is easy—and necessary. If it is agreed that our scientific goal is understanding and not prediction *per se*, then it follows that where one must choose between the alternatives, research should be oriented toward a limited increase in understanding rather than a great increase in predictability.

It is generally agreed that science has a consensual basis. Although an idiosyncratic perception may be more acute, it is not really understood until something is known of the process by which this greater accuracy is achieved, even if the perception still cannot be duplicated. If the discrimination basis remains a personal, even magical thing, then it provides no stuff for science. The discriminations may be used for practical ends but they offer no further leads toward the understanding that would allow encompassing more general and more varied features of our world.

A unique acuity has importance for understanding only if we are motivated or able to analyze its basis. If the phenomenon, when it occurs, is not studied, it remains simply a curiosity piece and not a datum of science. It is by this reasoning that individual evaluations are rejected as instruments of research. As a basis for hypothesis and "discovery" (Reichenbach, 1951), solitary perceptions of course are irreplaceable. Their status is questioned, however, when they are employed as sufficient data for proof or "justification."

If we are resigned, then, to the idea of combining judgments, how best may several evaluations be pooled so that the fairest representation of the subject's personality results? In one form or another, a whole host of methods have been addressed to this question for this is the familiar problem of how to form a composite judgment or group decision *in the absence of a criterion*[7]

---

[7] When a criterion is available, i.e., when we know precisely and for all time what it is we wish to predict, there are routine and effective ways (e.g., multiple

(Dingman & Guilford, 1954; Dunnette & Hoggatt, 1957; Horst, 1936; Jones, 1957; Kemeny, 1959; Lawshe & Nagle, 1952; Spearman, 1927; Wilks, 1938).

The presently proposed procedure for combining judgments is a simple and almost conventional one. It results in scores which are almost invariably quite equivalent to the scores issued by more complicated pooling schemes.[8] Because of this equivalence

---

correlation, discriminant function analysis) to combine in an optimal fashion the judgments of observers. Regrettably, such ultimate criteria do not exist in the study of personality. The aspiration of a science of personality is toward a complete specification of the personality properties of an individual. If we possessed this ultimate knowledge, it would be a simple matter to discover which judges most closely approach this idealized criterion. In the absence of a criterion, the combination of judges must be justified on other grounds.

[8] All the proposed techniques for combining judgments, with the exception of Kemeny's intriguing but untried method, reduce to suggestions that judges be weighted arbitrarily (and usually equally) in forming a composite or that judges be weighted in terms of their amount of agreement with each other. The presumption in this latter orientation is that the judge who agrees, on the whole, most highly with the other judges is likely to be most valid in his perceptions as well. The argument for the *a priori*, equal-weighting scheme is that in the absence of reliable knowledge that one judge is more accurate than another, the most parsimonious (and tactful) procedure is to accord equal status to each observer. Differential weighting procedures developed from a factor analytic rationale have been presented by Spearman (1927), Dingham and Guilford (1954) and Jones (1957). Equal weighting methods are described by Horst (1936), Wilks (1938) and Dunnette and Hoggatt (1957). It is important to recognize that differential weighting procedures become equal weighting procedures as inter-judge agreements become equal.

Clearly, there is sense to either alternative emphasis. On the one hand, it seems reasonable to give little credence to a judge with whom other judges agree but slightly. On the other side, by accenting the importance of modal evaluations, advanced and still unusual insights may fail to receive their due.

The simple method of combining judgments advocated here—of summing the Q-judgment values for a subject across all the contributing judges, where each judge has made his judgments with no knowledge of how the other judges have rated the subject—occupies a firmly intermediate position with regard to this issue. When observers differ among themselves in their extent of agreement with each other, the presently proposed method leads to differential weighting of the several judges. But the weighting coefficients issuing from the simple summation method are much less disproportionate than the weighting coefficients derived from factor analytic rationales. That is, although the simple summation method moves toward differential weighting, it does so less emphatically than other methods. Accordingly, a judge has to be severely discrepant with other observers before his contribution toward the group consensus is lessened significantly. And, of course, when judges agree among themselves, each judge contributes equally to the consensus.

For the algebraic statement of the weightings provided by the simple summation method, the reader is referred to Dunnette and Hoggatt (1957); for the more extreme,

and because of the convenience in practice of the procedure, the simple summation method of combining judgments has seemed the most reasonable one to employ.

Given, then, a reasonable method of combining judgments, what may be expected of this consensus? One characteristic of consensus scores is that they are almost invariably highly reliable if based upon more than two or three judges. The kind of reliability meant here is the correspondence to be expected when this consensus (or average) score is correlated with a consensus (or average) derived from *an equivalent set of judges.* That is, if we were to go to the trouble of gathering judgments from another set of judges sampled from the same judge population, derive a second consensus evaluation, and correlate this second consensus evaluation with the consensus evaluation derived from the first set of judges, the resulting correlation would be the reliability coefficient we speak of here. This correlation may be estimated conveniently by an application of the familiar Spearman-Brown prophecy formula and is a function of the number of judges and their intercorrelation.[9]

---

factor analytic weightings, Spearman (1927) or Stephenson's presentation (1953, pp. 174 ff) may be consulted.

It appears, then, that the simple summation method is a compromise which is never far from either of the points of view about combining judgments. At the same time, the method is most convenient to apply. This last is a not inconsiderable advantage for a truly equal weighting scheme and other differential weighting procedures involve formidable and delaying calculations.

[9]The Spearman-Brown formula is a fundamental formula in psychometrics and is used to infer the correlation between one composite and another, equivalently constructed composite. This correlation, the reliability of the composite, is given by the following formula:

$$\text{reliability of composite} = \frac{N \text{ (average inter-judge correlation)}}{1 + (N-1) \text{ (average inter-judge correlation)}}$$

where N is the number of judges contributing to the consensus.

Most recently, Rajaratnam, Cronbach and Gleser (1960) have extended the scope of the Spearman-Brown formula, which presumes all judges are equivalent, by showing that the formula applies even when judges are not presumed equal. The alternative, less assumptional rationale they employ is that a set of judges is simply a random sample from a universe of judges. This statistical development places a rational support under the otherwise puzzling and frequently obtained empirical finding that the Spearman-Brown formula estimates accurately the reliability of composite ratings even when its supposed assumptions are violated patently (Clark, 1935; Gordon, 1924; Remmers, 1931; Rosander, 1936).

Table 4 specifies the reliability of composite scores for varying numbers of judges and for varying degrees of average intercorrelations among judges, as estimated by the Spearman-Brown formula. From the table, it is clear that respectable reliabilities are feasible in typical research contexts.

TABLE 4

The Reliability of Consensus Evaluations as a Function of the Number and Intercorrelation of Judges

Average intercorrelation among judges	*Number of Judges*			
	2	3	5	8
.10	.18	.25	.36	.47
.30	.46	.56	.68	.77
.50	.67	.75	.83	.89
.70	.82	.88	.92	.95

Now let us consider this consensus score more closely for perhaps, although reliable, it is not the score we really desire. The consensus score reflects multiple, independently arrived-at perceptions. As a consensus, it shares the properties of all averages and has considerable sampling stability. As a consensus, it is also relatively independent of the individual raters who, in the aggregate but not in the particular, form the average. Individual raters may be added to or deleted from the consensus at random, without appreciably affecting the average for the group. It would appear then that we have met the requirements for observer-evaluations that were specified at the beginning of this section—the requirements of reliability and of autonomy of the observation index from a particular observer.

At the same time, because our chosen score is an average, simple psychometric logic argues quite convincingly that the consensus will cumulate validity disproportionately more rapidly than it will cumulate error. Idiosyncracies of observers, inattentions, and other observer flaws can be expected, in the main, to cancel each other and to let through the stubborn truth. The expectation of higher validity in the consensus is supported empirically almost universally in the research instances where the matter has been investigated (cf., e.g., Block, 1957b; Kelley & Fiske, 1951).

Although we have already considered the metascientific propriety of solitary observations, what is the likelihood that we are losing special insights which would be noted if we worked with the separated ratings of individual judges? The chance is quite small. This point is not widely recognized and consequently, it is probably worth the digression here to explain why the consensus does so much justice to separate and unique individual judgments.

A correlation coefficient can be computed between a judge's evaluation and the consensus which includes that judge's evaluations. The result is a part-whole correlation. It is obvious that as this part-whole correlation approaches unity, there is less and less possibility of a difference between the discriminations provided by the individual judge and the discriminations provided by the consensus which includes that judge.

Now, the part-whole correlation is a function of two factors, the number of judges and the intercorrelation of judges. Table 5 cites the part-whole correlations for the situations where the number of observers is two, three, five and eight, and their average intercorrelation (assumed to be equal) is zero, .50 and .71. These combinations probably bracket the various situations empirically encountered.

TABLE 5

PART-WHOLE CORRELATIONS UNDER VARIOUS CONDITIONS

Average Observer Intercorrelation	Number of Observer			
	2	3	5	8
.00	.71	.58	.45	.35
.50	.79	.71	.64	.59
.71	.87	.82	.78	.75

The conclusions to be drawn from this table is that, although the possibility yet exists that an individual judge will offer discriminations reliably different from those contained in the consensus (cf. McCornack, 1956), the part-whole correlations are so high there is little likelihood separate analyses would be worthwhile. With few or even a moderate number of judges, and even with relatively low inter-judge agreement, analysis of the consensus rating will discern almost all the relationships conceivably discernable by individual analyses. Only with larger numbers of judges than are usually used in research does a significant possibility emerge of differences in the results provided by the alternative approaches.[10] By and large, then the consensus judgement appears to be a fair and sensitive way of representing individual ratings. As already indicated, the consensus judgment has the additional happy faculty of being more valid, usually, than any of the individual judgments.

If observer-evaluations can be processed to achieve such desirable properties, why then have they been viewed with suspicion in the past? One reason is that attention was focused incorrectly and so good data appeared to be of poor quality. For example, much discouragement has been engendered by low intercorrelations among judges when, in fact, the consensus based upon these data would have quite satisfactory reliability. But often too, the consensual criterion has been abandoned from the outset, with evaluations being recorded by solitary judges.

Another disappointment has followed upon the recognition that perfecting interjudge agreement with regard to what are essentially scoring procedures has very immediate limits. That is, ratings of, for example, a Rorschach protocol are intrinsically limited by what a particular examiner happens to have written down. Much too much energy has gone into interpreting single, already filtered perceptions rather than in diversifying the basis for evaluation. If multiple, independent views of behavior are gathered and combined, however, we can almost guarantee a reliability and, in addition, increase the likelihood of finding the validities we seek.

Still another basis of dissatisfaction with observer-evaluations stems from the still frequently used conference method of diagnosing personality. In the conference method, a group of judges meet to discuss a subject and to formulate a decisive evaluation of the subject's personality. Now, it may be most informative (and it is certainly less lonely) for the judges to come together to compare and extend their personal formulations. In training or educational contexts, the conference method of formulating evaluations has a special value because the give and take of in-

---

[10] The reliability and generalizability of these differences would have to be assessed. Solely by chance, spotty differences can arise. It is important that chance fluctuations not be reified into fact.

formation proceeds easily in such settings. For research purposes, however, judgments issuing out of group interaction are inadvisable. Data that comes out of group debate tend to be influenced by all sorts of unspecifiable (or at least unreportable) factors such as the status or prestige of the various judges, their relative persuasiveness, the fortuitous interpersonal contagions that have an opportunity now to develop, and so on. Such data are confounded in unknown ways and their reliability cannot be assessed. Moreover, the *several or many* judges form only *one* group and so the reproducibility of conference judgments cannot be estimated. These complaints against this popular and congenial method would be but small annoyances if the method regularly demonstrated its larger validity. In fact, however, the little evidence on the matter strongly suggests that no predictive gains are contributed by the conference method (Kelly & Fiske, 1951). In achieving the pleasant circumstances of group discussion, it would appear that the participants in the conference method have only lessened the scientific merit of the information they initially possessed.

Improving the relevance of observer-evaluations. If observer-evaluations are truly important, and if they can be made objective and reliable, what can be done to increase the usefulness and incisiveness of the approach? It will be recalled that a fundamental criticism voiced against formalized observer-evaluations is that they are insensitive to the nuances an observer might wish to convey.

In responding to this criticism, we must first call attention to two essentially different ways in which observer-evaluations have been expressed in the past—by means of *ratings* and by means of *characterizations*. Ratings have predominated in the main stream of *psychological* research, while the characterological approach has prevailed in the *psychiatric* field. This very definite association of method with profession appears to come from the different emphases, the different kinds of understanding sought by the respective orientations.

Traditional psychological research into personality has taken a "variable-centered" approach and has employed methods and analyses appropriate to the specification of *the correlations among variables.* Personality evaluations, in this context, are stated within a "normative" frame of reference (Cattell, 1944), i.e., a subject is rated on a particular variable *vis-a-vis* a specified reference or "normative" group. A typical instance of a normative rating might be the assigning of "masculinity" or "conservatism" ratings, on a 5-point scale, to each of 100 military officers.

The normative way to the specification of personality is well-tested and understood. It provides data in a convenient and quantitative form, and it has not been unproductive. Presently, it continues to be the most frequently employed rating approach. For a thoughtful presentation and discussion of the normative rating method, the reader is referred to Guilford (1954, ch. 11).

The psychiatric emphasis (included under this heading are psychologists working in the realm of psychopathology) has been a "person-centered" one. The concern here has not been with separately considered variables and their separate sets of inter-relationships, but rather with the closer understanding of individuals.

The strongly held belief by proponents of the "person-centered" approach is that normative ratings operate *in vacuo* and for this reason are deficient. What is required is an *in vivo* description of an individual, a description which can convey that individual's "essence," his crucial characteristics and their intertwinings, the appositions and oppositions in his personality structure. Conventionally, psychiatrists have used "clinical formulations" in the implementation of this goal.

Phrased alternatively and a bit more formally, when a subject is intensively and prolongedly studied, the inter-relationships of the personality variables (in terms of which the evaluation is to be expressed) take on *system-qualities.* Certain couplings and contingent dependencies among variables are perceived by the observer as specifying the laws of personality governing this particular observed person. Because of the manifold patterns of covariation and contingency that have been observed, because of the *different systems* of personality functioning which seem to exist, it would follow that a method of personality evaluation is required that can encompass and then re-issue this kind of information. So runs the "person-centered" argument.

This argument has a fundamental validity. Certainly, the pattern of co-variation that characterizes one group of individuals may differ greatly from the covariance pattern that characterizes another "type" of person. However, in the implementation of this view—by means of case histories, "clinical formulations" and the like—this emphasis on personality *qua* system has lost much of its usefulness for the scientific sphere. It would seem that the "system" viewpoint has been espoused without a sense of the discipline it requires when its kind of information is to be used for research purposes. A major reason for the discrepancy between proposal and accomplishment here can be seen in a problem posed by language usage.

One of the absolute requirements of the scientific method is that a relevant basis for relevant comparisons be established. Without the opportunity of making comparisons, relationships cannot be sought. Consequently, investigatory procedures must guarantee comparability of evaluation if their results are to be respected.

Unfortunately, language usage in personality description is highly variable, both within and between personologists. Characterological sketches vary widely as to detail, comprehensiveness, length, and—most important—literary style. Consequently, comparison of "write-ups" of the same or of different subjects proves to be at best a tortuous, prolonged process. More usually, it is simply an unrealizable objective.

The criticism of non-comparability of language usage is of crucial importance. Personality evaluations, in which may be imbedded the most valuable of perceptions and insights, cannot function as research material given the inability to make comparisons. Disagreements may be suggested that are genuinely nonexistent; unanimity of opinion may be presumed which we are unable to recognize as deceptively based. Undoubtedly, many false notions presently exist because there has been no means to lay them low. We simply *must* be enabled to compare and contrast formulations of personality so that we can see where we agree and where we disagree.

Now, free descriptions of a subject can differ for two reasons: (1) differences in what is perceived or in the way behavior is analyzed and integrated, and (2) basically irrelevant differences in phrase-making or language style. We need to respect the first of these factors, but not the second, which operates to confuse the critical issues.

In practice, variegated phrase-making often reflects an orientation other than the one toward description, with which the observer presumably is concerned. Instead of employing variety of expression in the search for aptness of formulation, the observer may simply be expressing his personal need for unusualness or originality of expression. The urge toward personalizing one's communications is an understandable one and indeed is a tendency those sensitive to literary style will applaud. It is regrettable that the effort in this context is damaging to the overriding scientific purpose we serve. It must also be mentioned that sometimes the free description becomes a stagy vehicle aimed at literary effect (and the evaluator's enhancement), with only casual regard for the claims of truth. This kind of vanity too requires discouragement. The special possibilities of the "person-centered" approach go unrealized when accurate perceptions are communicated in capricious or histrionic ways.

One way in which free descriptions can be made comparable so that the substantive problems—the issues of concern—can be approached is by permitting a standard vocabulary—a constant set of variables—to be used and used in a standard way.

Although the normative rating method has been one kind of response to this requirement—it offers a standard set of variables which may be quite extensive in coverage—it cannot be employed directly if we are to respect the "person-centered" approach. Only in a cumbersome way and after proper planning can the data provided by the normative method be adapted for "person-centered" research. It is much easier to collect data directly in the form desired rather than process possibly inappropriate normative data after-the-fact.

And so it is by this chain of reasoning that an application of the Q-sort scaling procedure (Stephenson, 1953) is suggested as an appropriate, simple, and useful method for the complex person-centered description of an individual in a form suitable for quantitative, statistical evaluation and comparison.

The Q-sort method is an "ipsative" procedure (Cattell, 1944), i.e., the personality variables in the defined set are ordered or scaled relative to each other, with respect to a specified criterion and with a specific subject as the frame of reference. In the usual application, a set of personality variables are arranged in an order reflecting the relative "salience" of these variables *vis-a-vis* each other in characterizing a particular person. For example, the judge may be asked to assign *relative* ratings of "masculinity" and "conservatism" as these qualities apply to the person being described. Is "masculinity" a more crucial attribute of the subject than his "conservatism"? Or is the trait of "conservatism" more decisive than the trait of "masculinity" for an understanding of the person?

The ipsative Q-method provides "person-centered" data in numerical form, data which are analyzable in a variety of ways. Of special significance is the way the procedure permits expression by the assessor of how he sees the defined set of personality variables to be arranged within the person being characterized.

The remainder of this monograph is devoted to an exposition and discussion of what we have designated as the California Q-set (the CQ-set), a carefully selected and slowly evolved set of personality variables conjoined with a standard way of using these variables—our specific version of the Q-scaling procedure.

The purpose of the CQ-set is to provide a "Basic English" for clinical psychologists, psychiatrists, and personologists to use in their formulations of individual personalities. Ideally—and the set is not ideal—the items should permit the portrayal of any kind of psychopathology and of any kind of normality. Despite the constraints the method (any method) involves, the descriptions possible through the CQ-set should be perceived by the assessor as registering in a sufficient and sensitive manner his impression of the personality of the person being described. To the extent the set fails in this aspiration, to the extent it is deemed unable to reflect the discriminations and integrations of the observer, the method is to be judged deficient.

No claim is made here that the CQ-set represents an ultimate achievement or delineation of the necessary and sufficient facets in terms of which personality is to be understood. Rather, it is suggested that the CQ-set, by virtue of its initial rationale and developmental history, provides a broadly ranging and therefore widely useful language for personality description.

The CQ-set presently to be described is the product of more than seven years of effort. During this time, about fifty psychologists and psychiatrists have contributed to the method, a dozen or so studies of the technique and its applications have been completed, and its psychometric properties have been analyzed and adjusted.

It has seemed appropriate to bring all of this material together at the present time for several reasons:

a. The method has proven quite helpful in a number of studies. In its present form, it embodies a good deal of thought and experience and it seems likely that a number of psychologists and psychiatrists will find the method congruent with their own research requirements.

b. Interest already expressed in the technique has suggested the desirability of a statement at this time detailing its history, rationale, applications, and the cautions to be observed in its use.

c. Although the present version of the CQ-set is already broadly based, increased application of the procedure can be expected to result in valid suggestions for its improvement. Although the procedure is to remain stabilized for a period of some years, we should like to be able to incorporate accumulated improvements in a later revision of the method rather than prematurely consider the CQ-set as "frozen" into its final form. With this perspective on the rationale and aspirations underlying the CQ-procedure, we may consider the effort now in more detail.

Chapter III

STEPHENSON'S ORIENTATIONS TOWARD
Q-SET CONSTRUCTION

I F we are going to restrict ourselves to a basic vocabulary, it is clear we should choose our words most carefully.
We shall be unable to rise above the restrictions set by our initially agreed-upon language.

It was because of this recognition that most of the effort in
developing the CQ-set has been concentrated on establishing a
"good" set of personality variables. With full awareness that we
are limited and contained in our generalizations as a function of
the variables finally selected, the expectation has been that this
constraint could be reduced greatly by care and by the correc-
tions which can come only from experience. Moreover, in the
present state of psychological investigation, it was felt that any
insufficiencies in the item set developed would prove slight compared to other inadequacies in contemporary research method.
We shall return later to this last point.

With agreement on the primacy of the requirement of a *comprehensive* set of personality items, how to begin? What are the
rules to follow in insuring achievement of this desideratum?

As it turns out, there is no agreed-upon set of rules available
in the literature to guide us along our way. Literally, the only
remarks on the fundamental problem of item *content* are those by
Stephenson, the ingenious innovator, vigorous proponent and
almost solitary expositor of the Q-method. Regrettably, his stated
views, for our present purposes, do not provide a satisfactory
rationale for the construction of a set of Q-items. If Stephenson's
book (1953) is taken as his most definitive statement on the
matter, we find three methods of Q-set construction described
therein.

1. According to Stephenson, having first defined a domain or universe of intended coverage, one may simply enumerate a list of variables or items deemed appropriate and employ these as a "Q-sample." For example, an experimenter might have decided to investigate the field of masculinity-femininity. By this first method of Stephenson, the investigator would simply make up and use a batch of statements that, in his view, were related to the *masculinity-feminity* domain.

However, this attractively simple approach, when casually embarked upon, can lead to casual and simplistic results. There is the great likelihood that *the results obtained by means of a Q-set so established are idiosyncratic functions of the unspecified basis for originally including items.* Items representative of a domain for one investigator might not be judged representative by other investigators. Because of the difficulty in interpretation of results thus achieved, this historically first method lost favor in Stephenson's eyes, and a more objective—if tedious— procedure was submitted. Nevertheless, a number of users of the Q-sort method have employed this method of Q-set construction, with its attendant dangers of solipsism.

2. The second method proposed by Stephenson for developing Q-sets requires operational specification of the universe of interest. *All* the statements that, by some operational criterion, fall within the chosen domain are first collected. For example, in a study of Jungian types, Stephenson was able to aggregate some 2000 statements made by Jung in discussing introverts and extroverts. From this large and unwieldy universe were selected, strictly at random, samples of items which then served as the Q-sets to be used in subsequent research.

The advantages of this orientation are several. The entire procedure is specifiable and consequently reproducible. The Q-sets derived are truly representative of the delimited universe and, as a corollary, comparable Q-sets are readily achieved by successive sampling from this universe. This is the method that Hilden (1954; 1958) has employed in his Q-work.

The reason why this method has not especially taken hold, aside from the indefinitely extended labors that collecting an item-universe will often entail, is that it fails to consider the nature of the universe it samples. *The operations by means of which a universe is made concrete provide no guarantee that the aggregation so resulting will be a proper expression of the underlying (and abstractly defined) universe.* Thus, there may be extreme redundancies in coverage of certain portions of the domain, and great territories of experience or personality that are scarcely alluded to. Random sampling from an operationally specified universe of unknown bias offers no assurance of an ultimate representativeness of coverage.

3. The third Stephenson proposal for constructing Q-sets represents a radical extension of his initial logic. This last method—of "structured" Q-items—has not proven acceptable to psychologists, at least as it has been advocated by Stephenson. Aside from the initial studies by him in illustration of the method, no other applications have appeared in the literature.

By means of a "structured" Q-set, Stephenson would have the Q-items embody an analysis of variance design in two or three (but not many more) dimensions. The results emerging from variance analysis of a structured Q-sample would, in principle, bear upon the *interactions* of the independent variables, matters of great importance to personality theory and practice. In addition, the variance design, by specifying the nature and number of the items required to fill its various cells, offers a rationale for item selection which escapes the dangers of undue weighting of unknown factors. This characterization of the method can be given life by an example taken from Stephenson (1953, p. 69ff).

Out of Jung's type psychology, Stephenson identified three main concepts—the orientations of *introversion* or *extroversion*, the *conscious-unconscious* distinction (i.e., awareness or unawareness of the driving principle underlying one's behavior) and third, the various "functions"—of *thinking, feeling, sensation,* and *intuition.* If this triumvirate is regarded as three independent variables, a 2 x 2 x 4 design may be permutated. Each possible combination of these concepts thus is posited to exist and each of these possibilities can be "clothe[d] . . . with statements. . . . We merely take assertations by Jung which comport with these combinations, one statement to each combination. Thus, Jung's statement 'ready to sink a battleship or to amputate a leg' would fit into (the *extroversion-conscious-feeling* category); 'quietly sensual' into (the *introversion-unconscious sensation* cell)" (1953, p. 69-70), and so on until each of the combinations has a statement assigned to it. The design may then be replicated by finding additional sets of statements to fit the available categories.

The full set of structured items is sorted in the usual manner, the resulting scale values for each item being entered as scores into the appropriate cell of the design. Presumably, analysis of variance of these values could then indicate, for example, that an individual is consciously an extrovert but unconsciously an introvert, and so on.

Such findings, if one could have faith in them, would be important indeed and the structured Q-set would represent a distinguished advance in personality methodology. Unfortunately, we cannot have this confidence, and for reasons intrinsic to the method.

Although the method provides, from the design combinations, an orderly if limited basis for item-selection, in practice it is a most ambiguous task to find items appropriate to specific cells, for by what criteria shall items be assigned? Properly attempted, the research effort involved in item search and in the required item justifications is formidable and with no assurance of the possibility of success at its end. If, on the other hand, statements are assigned imperially to cells, the research resulting simply is not convincing.

Stephenson's structured sample for Jung's theory is presented in full in his book (1953, pp. 83-85), presumably as a positive instance of the method. The reader interested in this last approach by Stephenson is advised to consult this illustrative set of items. To most psychologists, it seems that the statements are only obscurely related, if at all, to the categories they nominally represent. On what basis, for example, can the items, "Impulsive and unrestrained," "A 'prophet,'" "Is underestimated and misunderstood," all be assigned to the same category; *introversion-unconscious-intuition?* What reasoning underlies the assignment of the items "Ponderous" and "Unreasonable" to the *extroversion-conscious-feeling* cell? Clearly, the reproducibility by other

psychologists of the classification of items would be extremely low
—a devastating defect in the approach.

In addition to the above criticism, Cronbach and Gleser (1954)
in an extended review of the Stephenson book call attention to a
number of other weaknesses in the structured sample approach.
The interested reader may wish to refer to their remarks.

And so, Stephenson's most ambitious method for selecting
Q-items has failed of acceptance also. Aside from a few "practical considerations" to be respected in establishing Q-sets—considerations such as understandability, conciseness and so on—
this is all that Stephenson has said on this central feature of his
total technique. Indeed, he takes at times an impatient, almost
detached attitude toward the whole problem. He is content with
a "rough-and-ready universe of statements" from which, with "a
certain art" and with "certain precautions," a sample "suitable to
the needs of a particular study" is compiled (1953, pp. 76-78).
Especially should it be noted that Stephenson considers it "a mistake to regard a sample as a standardized set or *test* of statements. . . ." (1953, p. 77)—a view contrary to the orientation of
the present work.

We have discussed Stephenson's suggestions for selecting Q-
items at such length for two reasons. First, he holds a position
as primary protagonist of the method. Beyond his recommendations, there are no alternative guides in the literature.[11] And
second, our disagreements with the Stephenson suggestions in
effect shaped the rationale at which we finally arrived in our own
Q-set construction.

---

[11] In brief remarks, Cronbach (1953) and Goodling and Guthrie (1956) have
separately offered the suggestions, out of orthodox test construction practice, that
Q-items show variance across subjects and be equated with respect to their average
degree of social desirability. The special—and fundamental—problem of Q-item
content has been discussed only by Stephenson.

Chapter IV

CONSTRUCTING THE CALIFORNIA Q-SET

P<small>RIOR</small> to the explicit intention of developing a comprehensive and widely applicable Q-set for use by psychologists and psychiatrists, the writer had been active in a number of other Q-studies (1952a; 1954; 1955a). In late 1952, a memorandum was prepared which presented the case for the Q-sort procedure as a means of codifying personality formulations in an assessment setting (Block, 1952b). This memorandum led to the preparation[12] of a Q-set for use by assessors in a study of Air Force officers (MacKinnon *et al.* 1958). In many respects, this early deck of IPAR Q-items may be considered a precursor of the CQ-set for the rapidly apparent capabilities of this IPAR collection of items served to encourage the larger effort to develop an exhaustive and more generally useful Q-set.

With recognition of the contribution a competent set of Q-items could make, the enterprise began. Some 90 personality variables were expressed in item form, aiming at comprehensive coverage of the personality domain as viewed by contemporary clinicians. Many of these items were taken or adapted from the earlier IPAR set. This initial assembly of variables was of course an unspecifiable function of the writer's personal theoretical preferences.

The principles employed in writing CQ-items were several:

1) Each item was written in a theoretically neutral form. Although a psycho-dynamic orientation frankly underlies the CQ-set, the items themselves presumably are committed to no special theoretical viewpoint. No CQ-item embodies a concept linked exclusively to one theoretical orientation and so the personality

---

[12] In conjunction with Robert E. Harris and assisted by other members of the IPAR staff.

formulations built up by the CQ-elements should be compatible with any of the several viewpoints about personality.

2) Each item was written to suggest a continuum, rather than to have either-or implications. It was intended that the salience or decisiveness of an item would be expressed by its placement rather than directly by its wording; e.g., "is distrustful of people in general" would imply paranoia when placed as positively salient.

3) Each item was written to express single psychological "elements" to avoid the equivocality engendered by "double-barrelled" phrasings. For example, the statement "is talkative and self-assured" is a poor item in that the subject may be talkative but not self-assured, or self-assured but not talkative. Partitioning such items into their constituent elements eliminates what can be a formidable problem for the sorter while still permitting complex conjunctions of elements to be expressed.

4) An effort was made to include only variables that were conceptually independent of each other, even if these items proved to be functionally related in the usual case. By conceptual independence is meant that the psychological sense of each item could not be coordinated to or derived from the psychological sense of any other item or conjunction of items.

Of course, in the present state of our knowledge and analysis of the personality domain, this principle can be followed only as an ideal, not with the assurance of achievement. Experience with and psychometric analyses of provisional item-sets can move us a long way toward the goal, however. The CQ-set, initiated with the orientation of conceptual requiredness for each item, has in its present form presumably profited a great deal from the knowledge afforded by its earlier versions.

5) Related to the preceding emphasis on the conceptual independence of items is the attitude taken with respect to a certain redundancy of statements. The presence of empirical correlation among items may not be totally undesirable. While a certain wastefulness of effort is suggested where two items are known to correlate appreciably, it may be worthwhile to carry along this overlap in order to preserve the possibility of expressing in the Q-sort those very crucial instances of personality

configurations where the usual correlation does *not* exist. Thus, *rigidity* and *conservatism* may be expected to correlate fairly well in most subject populations, but certainly not perfectly. It is important to be able to describe the individual with the one characteristic but not the other for there are instances where a conventional relationship fails to hold. In order to express the many exceptions to usual correlation, exceptions which quite properly may crystallize and determine an entire personality formulation, it is desirable to include related (but not equivalent— cf. point 3, above) variables.

Obviously, careful and consensual value judgments are required in implementing this respect for inconsistencies in syndromes. The success or utility of this particular emphasis, as it has affected the developing CQ-set, may better be evaluated later in this monograph, and best after actual use of the instrument. For the present, we wish simply to note that this orientation has guided the CQ-set since its inception.

6) A further facet of the redundancy problem arises from the recognition that, often enough, logical or verbal opposites are not necessarily psychological opposites. For example, *submission* is the verbal opposite of *dominance*. Yet there exists a kind of person for whom both of these variables are positively salient simultaneously—the so-called "authoritarian-submissive personality."

As another illustration, an item on *impulsivity* does not displace an item on *constriction* if we are to be able to describe the individual who is characteristically inconsistent in his pattern of impulse-control.

Or, a personality variable may have a number of "opposites." A person who is *not* "self-abasing" may be "self-accepting" or he may be "critical of others."

If we are to be able to map the nuances and complexities of personality by mere words—words which have a sometime relation to other words—then an additional component of redundancy must be incorporated into the Q-set to cope with these equivocal possibilities.

7) A final concern was to minimize the degree of value judgment in the judges' descriptions of subjects. In principle, professional observers should be dispassionate in their perceptions;

in reality, their frailties are ever-present. One way to prevent value judgments from dominating the descriptive function of a judge is to provide him with a language which already has excluded values from consideration. Toward this end, effort was made to compose items in a neutral and unevaluative form. Necessarily, however, a number of the variables selected for inclusion in the CQ-set prove to carry positive implications for the subject's character and a number clearly refer to negative or undesirable properties of personality. These "evaluative" items are unavoidable in the sense that they are *conceptually required* if a comprehensive description is to be offered. As judged by raters, neutral, positive and negative items exist in the CQ-set in the ratio, approximately, of 2:1:1.

In usage, the positive and negative CQ-items do not appear to have been especially susceptible to unfortunate stereotype effects. Within the set of positive or negative items, there is appreciable psychological heterogeneity. A global, undifferentiated adulation or condemnation of a subject therefore is readily identified by its caricature of psychological health or disorder.

It cannot be claimed that in all regards the principles of Q-set construction just enunciated were followed with complete success. Undoubtedly, certain CQ-items can be interpreted ambiguously or as double-barreled. By some psychologists, the CQ-variables still may be viewed as jargon-laden. We have—deliberately—mixed levels of interference and merged inter- and intra-personal orientations and for some purposes or for some partisan inclinations, such a decision may be unacceptable. The balance struck on redundancy is also open to question. We may have excised as excessively redundant items which, for certain purposes, would provide the fine discriminations desired or it may be argued that too much redundancy still remains.

We are not backing off from a respect for the labors involved in forming and testing the CQ-items. Rather, we are recognizing that, in the nature of our imperfect world, there exist no criteria by which we may judge the extent to which these principles of item-writing are satisfied. Assurances certainly may be offered, because the CQ-items were developed employing a broad base of psychological and psychiatric opinion, and because of the opportunity provided by earlier usages to study and refine the CQ-variables, that very many difficulties and insufficiencies in the CQ-set have been eliminated. We may only suggest—*not* assure—that a broad spectrum of assessment psychologists and psychiatrists will find the resulting version useful and versatile. Now, to historical details.

Evolving the CQ-set, Form I. The ninety items assembled out of the foregoing orientation constituted a starting point. This provisional set was then the focus of intensive and prolonged discussions with two other psychologists[13] and a psychoanalyst.[14] In some sixty hours of meetings, each item was taken up in turn and discussed with respect to its clarity, its psychological importance and its implications for the sufficiency of the total Q-deck.

The task of achieving clarity was simply an editing job. The guiding editorial principles here were several—conciseness where possible, amplifications where judged necessary, elimination of unrequired or multiply-understood professional jargon, item phrasings that stayed within the conceived universe of discourse (e.g., high metaphors were ruled out).

The psychological importance of an item was the judgment, by consensus after discussion, of the information value and general relevance of the particular item in describing personality. By virtue of the consensual basis for decision on this property of items, the initially offered collection of items took its first step away from idiosyncratic emphasis toward the goal of a wider acceptability and usefulness.

As items were reworked and rejudged, they became familiar in meaning and in capability. The third and most decisive criterion then proved usable, namely, were the Q-items—now clear and agreed to be important—sufficient in themselves or in *combination* to encompass the full range of personality constellations?

No analytical method for testing the adequacy of the Q-set of course existed for the simple reason there exists no exhaustively systematic and widely accepted conceptualization of personality. And so an empirical effort was made by members of the group to

---

13 Jeanne H. Block and Virginia Patterson.
14 Don D. Jackson.

find weaknesses in the item sample. Illustrations out of experience and hypothetical, albeit possible, instances were invoked to embarrass the descriptive capabilities of the Q-set as it existed at that temporal point.

Whenever it was judged that a gap or inadequacy had been noted in the Q-set, whenever some facet of personality judged important proved unexpressable fairly by an existing item or *some conjunction of existing items,* then suitable item revisions were made or an appropriate item was written and added to the Q-set.

The emphasis on the descriptive possibilities residing in *conjunctions* of Q-items is an important strategy to note. Thus, the item "is fatherly" was not included in the CQ-set for the reason that a conception of "fatherliness" could be expressed by conjoining such CQ-items as "Is turned to for advice and reassurance," "Is protective of those close to him," "Behaves in a masculine style and manner," "Is calm, relaxed in manner," "Has warmth; has the capacity for close relationships; compassionate," and others. Very many would-be items could be excluded when evaluated against the meaning of a *constellation* of existing items.

After the initial group had deliberated extensively and offered its item choices, the resultant Q-set was submitted to the group of clinical psychologists then (1953) at the Langley Porter Clinic.[15] In a series of a half-dozen seminars, the Q-items were discussed again with this new group. And again, the desiderata toward which discussion was oriented were defined as clarity, importance, and sufficiency. Appreciable change in the Q-set came out of these meetings, for the challenge to the group to find personality-relevant items not already included was taken up with vigor.

With the completion of this second set of discussions, it was decided to "freeze" the Q-set as it stood at that point. The original collection of items had been broadened considerably in perspective and acceptability, a benefit accruing from the multi-

---

[15] Among those on the staff at the time, and cooperating in this endeavor, I can recall R. E. Harris, Bernard Apfelbaum, Betty Kalis, Albert Shapiro, Elaine Simpson, John Starkweather, and Leon Witebsky.

ple viewpoints brought to bear upon it. It seemed opportune to test the Q-set's research utility and its psychometric properties. Accordingly, for a 14-month period, beginning in July 1953, the revised array of now 108 items, identified as the CQ-set, Form I, was used without further change in several researches.

Evolving the CQ-set, Form II. In August of 1954, the CQ-set, Form I was revised. In the course of employing Form I, various psychologists had offered additional suggestions for improvement of the item-set, suggestions growing out of actual research or teaching experience with the procedure.[16] The suggestions were a fundamental resource in guiding the revision made at this time.

As a most valuable by-product of a study employing the CQ-set, Form I to study psychiatrists' conceptions of the schizophrenogenic parent (Jackson, J. Block, J.H. Block, & Patterson, 1958), remarks on the CQ-set were available from five of the participating psychiatrists. These memoranda were surveyed as another source of instruction for the revision.

A final basis for directing the revision came from the results of an analysis of 240 applications of Form I in a study reported elsewhere (J. H. Block, Patterson, J. Block, & Jackson, 1958). The primary emphasis of this psychometric analysis was to eliminate uninformative items. Dispersions for each item were calculated in order to find items showing little variation over a wide range of subjects. Such items convey little differential information. If the small dispersion for an item was judged as an intrinsic property of that item and as *not* due to the special characteristics of the subject sample providing the data, then that item was eliminated from the revision.

A secondary psychometric consideration affecting the revision was the extent of correlation inspectionally noted as existing among items. Computational facilities did not at the time permit generation of the complete item covariance matrix but selected

---

[16] My colleague, Harrison G. Gough, at the Institute of Personality Assessment and Research, University of California, provided some especially incisive recommendations for the revision. Sustaining their earlier interest in the venture and constructively criticizing Form I were Jeanne Block and Robert E. Harris. Shirley Hecht, Mary Rauch, Paul Petersen and Donald C. Woodworth also contributed helpful suggestions.

correlations between various obviously related items were computed to see if excessive redundancy was present.

The CQ-set, Form II, benefiting as it did from additional intelligences and returns from experience, could properly be said to be another step along in the direction of achieving consensual utility—a descriptive capability sufficiently versatile to permit personality formulations by a wide range of psychodynamically oriented observers.

The CQ-set, Form II consisted of 115 items and was used from August 1954 until March 1957, when Form III, the present version of the CQ-set, replaced it. During this time, Form II achieved fairly intensive usage, being employed in assessment programs and research at the Institute of Personality Assessment and Research, at Vassar, at Minnesota, and in the Veterans Administration. Form II was also used as a teaching device in courses at the University of California.

Evolving the CQ-set, Form III. In the Fall of 1956, a tentative revision of Form II of the CQ-set was prepared, incorporating the suggestions accumulated from users in the preceding two years. This tentative revision provided the content of a series of weekly meetings held at the Institute of Human Development (formerly the Institute of Child Welfare) during the Winter and Spring of 1956-57. At these meetings the group discussed each of the Q-items, evaluating them, singly and in conjunction, against the criteria described earlier. The group participating was most helpful, contributing a number of refinements to the item set.[17]

Concomitant with this further refinement of the Q-set through further discussion, an extensive psychometric analysis of the properties of the items in Form I and II was carried through. An IBM Model 701 digital computer recently had become available. Its resources were employed to generate for each item its mean, dispersion and correlation with all other items in each of four separate (and quite different) samples.

The 108 items in the CQ-set, Form I were intercorrelated, the

---

[17] For their aid and insights, I am pleased to record my debt here to Jean Walker Macfarlane, Marjorie Honzik, Betty Kalis, Edith Katten, Norman Livson, and Irene Rosenthal.

data being derived from a sample of 40 mothers of psychiatrically-disturbed children and, as a separate matrix, from a sample of 40 fathers of these psychiatrically-disturbed children.

The 115 items in the CQ-set, Form II were intercorrelated, the data here coming from Q-descriptions of a sample of 50 middle-aged Vassar graduates and, as a separate matrix, from a sample of 70 male applicants to medical school.

These four matrices were examined in order to identify uninformative items, i.e., items correlating too highly with other items in the set. In this scanning for redundancy, it was required that the wastefully high correlation between two items had to exist in more than one of the matrices. This condition was set as a safeguard against the premature conclusion that two items were functionally equivalent. If two items did not correlate highly in *each* of the different samples, this could only mean that different patterns of item covariation existed in the several groups. The decision in these instances was that such a finding needed to be respected, even at the cost of including an item that perhaps even usually was redundant.[18]

Another criterion employed in evaluating the properties of the Q-set at this time was that the *average* inter-person correlation within each sample be low, of the order of .10 or .15, with a *continuous* distribution of inter-person correlation.[19] As the average inter-person correlation *within* a sample increases, less discrimination *among* the individuals being correlated is possible. A relatively high average inter-person correlation legitimately may exist, when the sample clearly is a homogeneous one. In a sample judged to be heterogeneous in nature, however, a high average inter-person *r* can arise only when certain items are placed equivalently for all individuals. Such items are known as

---

[18] Because the measurement properties of CQ-items vary markedly as a function of the sample being studied, data on the properties of the CQ-items—their means, standard deviations, and R-type factor loadings—are not reported here.

[19] The requirement of a continuous distribution of inter-person correlations was invoked to guarantee that the *average* was an appropriate descriptive measure to consider. With a discontinuous distribution consisting of very high positive and very high negative inter-person *r*'s, an average close to zero could still be found. For obvious reasons, a low average in this context would be misleading.

"universals" because they apply to all people. "Universal" items introduce no special bias if the data are analyzed properly but they are wasteful since they are useless as discriminators. When these items of little variance in several samples were found, they were either eliminated or restated in an effort to enhance their potential for genuine variance.

With the parallel completion of the psychometric analysis and the discussion of items, Form III of the CQ-set was formalized. Form III contains 100 Q-items, listed in Table 1 and, for convenience, as Appendix A, and is the current descriptive set. Because of the several considered revisions and pre-testing the technique has undergone since its inception, no change of the CQ-set, Form III is imminent. At some future time, when the usefulness and deficiencies of the method in its present version have been tested, another revision may seem in order.

At this writing, the CQ-set, Form III is being employed in research projects at the Institute of Personality Assessment and Research, at the Institute of Human Development, in the Veterans Administration, at the Palo Alto Medical Research Foundation, in various projects of the State of California, at the University of California Medical School, as a teaching device at the University of California and in a number of individual researches at universities, medical schools and hospitals in this country.

Chapter V

EVALUATION OF THE CQ-ITEMS

As we have noted earlier, if a common language is to be substituted for individual styles of expression, some assurances are required that the vocabulary and the grammar of the imposed language are sufficient for its purpose. Failing this requirement, the effort is properly rejected. Given some confidence that the Q-method is basically appropriate, the unquestionable appeal of uniquely-phrased expression may, albeit wistfully, be abandoned for many purposes.

Questions of grammar and form we leave until the next chapter. For the present we deal with the question of vocabulary, namely: Are the presently-offered CQ-items rich enough, in the aggregate, to accomplish sufficiently well their descriptive purpose? What are the constraints imposed upon the perceptive observer when he is forced to express himself by means of—and only by means of—the items which happen to be in the CQ-set?

Let it be admitted, immediately and bluntly, that there *are* constraints. Indeed, constraints, restrictions, arbitrary exclusions, over-simplifications, and so on are inherent in the scientific enterprise. Our general countering argument to the complaint of constraint must build its case by claims of productivity for the method. If this claim is supported, the constraints appear acceptable, and what is excluded is, by this pragmatic criterion, not fundamental. And now, to the particulars—of criticism and rejoinder.

1. A frequent criticism of the Q-sort method is that the results obtained by its application are a function of the *particular* Q-set employed. With another Q-set, the relationships might be very different. If the instrument of observation, by its happenstance properties, controls decisively and restrictively the events re-

corded, one can have little faith in the results offered out of the method. To change the Q-set will mean the findings issuing through the Q-set will change as well.

This criticism can well be true and when true may well be devastating. Admittedly, a Q-set assembled without care or sophistication may have very powerful, special, and unspecifiable emphases. There may be massive redundancies or spectacular lacunae to affect the tilt of relationships perceived through the Q-set.

The criticism here is really the criticism leveled against the first two Stephenson orientations toward Q-set construction (cf. Ch. III). The obvious and quite sufficient response to this danger of special bias in the Q-set is simply to employ a consensual basis for item-selection. This has been the evolutionary course the CQ-set has taken, and certainly the scope of the items has been greatly extended in the process. At one time or another, over 50 professional persons of diverse orientations have contributed their suggestions to the set, suggestions stemming from their theoretical predispositions and suggestions evolving out of actual use of the item-set. If there is a bias in the CQ-set, it is a bias that has survived this rather large number of screenings. A bias so resistant to cancellation represents, if not a truth, at least a widely held belief among professional observers that the bias is to be desired. Such a belief cannot be challenged, at least not within the framework set by our initial aspiration, namely, to provide a procedure whereby contemporary psychodynamically-oriented observers could express sensitively their formulations of personality.

Given our defined goal, the criterion of achievement of this goal becomes consensual agreement by the population of professionals who would be potential users of the CQ-set. If the item set were to pass inspection by *all* members of this large and inaccessible population, then perfection would be upon us. In this real world, we have employed a sample of 50 observers as contributors to and definers of the CQ-set. The question thus becomes: is this a large enough number, or would another sample of 50 clinicians evolve a Q-set with appreciably different *functional properties?*

Of course, an independently constructed Q-set would be un-likely to duplicate *exactly* any existing items in our CQ-set. Nevertheless, *the functional relationships educed by the one Q-set can be expected to be very similar to the functional relationships appearing via the other Q-set.* There is both logic and empirical evidence behind this rather strong assertion.

The logical argument comes by analogy out of psychometrics. It is well recognized that an average score is a more valid indicator of the domain it represents than are any of the constituent scores on which the average is based. Translating this observation to the present context, it would follow that the *consensually evolved* Q-set is more valid in its coverage of its intended domain than would be Q-sets elaborated by any *one* of the contributing observers.

Now, this analogy is not to be taken at face value, for the CQ-set was evolved not by an averaging procedure but rather by *successive* screenings of the items. This lack of independence perhaps means early opinions were more influential in determining the CQ-variables than later ones despite the constant directive to users and revisors of the item-set to introduce variables not yet specified. Nevertheless, it is fair to expect that widening the base of contributions to a Q-set will be a powerful method of attaining convergence upon a broadly useful assemblages of variables.

Some empirical support for the contention that the functional distinctions made by one broadly-based Q-set will not differ appreciably from the functional distinctions made by a second broadly-based Q-set comes from an IPAR study of several years ago, conducted by the writer. In this experiment, two quite different Q-decks were employed by the same raters with reference to the same social objects. The similarities and differences among the subjects as separately reflected by the two Q-sets were evaluated two different ways and it was shown that psychologically equivalent results were available with either of the Q-decks. A more detailed description of this study is to be found in Appendix C.

Neither of the two Q-decks employed in this study were CQ-sets, and indeed one of these Q-sets was—quite deliberately—very casually constructed. The finding of functional identity in this experiment where great disparity existed in the way in which the contrasted Q-sets were constructed is surely suggestive. We are entitled to expect that in more considered circumstances, where alternative groups of profesionals were involved and oriented toward the same goal, that a functional interchange-ability of Q-sets will result. Accordingly, we might as well settle upon one widely ranging set of Q-variables that will fit the needs of many researchers. Prosaic multiplication of Q-sets *ad libitum* will simply add confusion. By fixing upon one "good" set for widespread use, the interchange and comparison of information is made easy.

2. Another criticism voiced against the CQ-set is that the observer is constrained in the number of discriminations he is enabled to make. There are, it is argued, many more facets to personality than the CQ-set (any Q-set) can express.

Three different rejoinders apply to this contention. The first countering argument is a numerical one, the second justification introduces considerations of relativism, and the last suggests a compromise when this criticism is most passionately held.

a) It is possible to compute the number of different ways in which the 100 items in the CQ-set can be arranged into the designated nine categories which have become standard. This number proves to be 6.45×10^{85}, an incredibly large figure. We should note that in computing this number of possible item-constellations, we have been forced to presume independence in placement of each of these items and this assumption we know to be incorrect. By how much, it is difficult to say, for estimates of item-covariation quite properly vary greatly from sample to sample. But reduce the above figure by a factor of 10 or 100 or a million or a hundred million and we are still left with an immensely large array of different item configurations. As reflected by the number of permutations and combinations available to the user of the CQ-set, it would seem that a sufficient number of discrimination possibilities exists if the judge can use them reliably.

b) The response of relativism makes a simple if disputatious claim, namely, that the constraints entailed by the use of the CQ-set are slight relative to the constraints imposed on personality research elsewhere and by other methods. When one considers the low reliability of so many experimental procedures in psychology, when one recollects the fallibility of criterion measures or of diagnosis, it would seem that the constraints on discrimination imposed by the CQ-set in a research setting would *not* be the weakest link in the inferential chain. This is not to say that limitations of the CQ-set are unimportant and do not attenuate truth. It is only to suggest that the reliability and multiplicity of the discriminations afforded by the CQ-set indicate it is already a decent instrument. The research resources available for methodological improvement might more profitably be expended on other features of the total research enterprise.

c) There inevitably will arise circumstances where a description solely in terms of CQ-items will be inadequate. At such times, a freely-written characterization of the subject will be desirable in order to convey the information and perceptions which would otherwise be abandoned. It is important, however, in studies which at the outset have chosen to employ the CQ-procedure, that this option be exercised *in addition to rather than instead of* a CQ-sort. By employing both procedures, judges need feel no sense of loss, for the contribution of both approaches is preserved. There is extra effort required, but this is the cost of conviction—the conviction that the free description (or for that matter, the CQ-set) attains a goal not achievable otherwise.

3. Still another remark made against the CQ-set concerns itself with the meaning and interpretability of the items used. Although the primary purpose of the Q-approach is to standardize a language so that comparability of description becomes possible, perhaps the standard language will still not be used in equivalent ways. The item "is aggressive" (which is *not* included in the CQ-set) might be interpreted by one observer in terms of *hostile tendencies*, and by another as simply a way of characterizing *assertiveness*.

To this problem of interpretation, we first call attention to the prolonged and careful evolution of item phrasing, as described earlier. The meaning of each item is, we believe, more direct and unequivocal than would usually be the case with rapid item construction. The manifest or genotypical level which an item is intended to reflect is clearly indicated. Jargon is minimized. Where an item is phrased alternatively or is elaborated, care was taken that these extensions be consonant with each other. So, it seems fair to say that such problems of interpretability as could be anticipated were dealt with.

Nevertheless, in actual usage, the interpretability problem may still arise. Different observers may come with radically different language backgrounds, conventions, emphases, and so on. One very fruitful technique we have employed in these instances is to have the several observers calibrate themselves by describing the same subject. As part of the preliminaries to a research where the CQ-set is to be used, calibration sessions are very important, for they provide the opportunity, after the CQ-set has been applied, of discussion among the observers. The discrepant observers can here come to know the bases of disagreement and can thus separate out such disagreement as is due to genuine difference in evaluation from unwanted discrepancies due to differing inter-pretations of items. A series of calibration sessions can do much to converge an initially disparate set of observers.

There is still the possibility that, although within a specific research the Q-set users may have attuned themselves to each other, the usages evolved may differ from the item-interpretations held elsewhere or in general. In order to help eliminate this contingency or at least provide a means of estimating its effect, Appendices D through F present CQ-set descriptions of the op-timally adjusted person, the male paranoid and the female hysteric.

Each of these CQ-descriptions is an average Q-sort derived from the CQ-sets independently offered by 9 different psycholo-gists. Associated with each of these "standard" descriptions is (1) a statement of the reproducibility of that composite and (2) an estimate of the correlation to be expected between an individual's independently formulated CQ-description of that syndrome or personality and the consensus description reported in the appen-dix. In order to form this estimate, it was necessary to make the assumption that the individual newly offering his Q-description is of a competence equal to those originally contributing to the consensus.

New users of the CQ-set can refer their own Q-descriptions of these conceptual diagnostic entities to these "standards," thus checking upon the communality of their perceptions.

The consensus descriptions in these appendices have another function to serve. The arguments so far for the CQ-set have been relatively recondite ones. We have called attention to the desirability of some such device, entered into detail as to how and why the CQ-set evolved as it did, and countered—still at an abstract level—criticisms that have been leveled against the method.

But the proof of the approach lies in its performance. And its performance is judged essentially by how fittingly the CQ-descriptions seem to portray their intended objects. The reader still personally unfamiliar with the workings of the CQ-set may wish to evaluate the adequacy of the descriptions in these appendices against his own understanding of the concepts or personalities described, to see how well they mesh.

4. A final concern voiced in regard to the CQ-set has to do with the problem of behavioral levels and clinical inference. Although many of the CQ-items require of the judge only that he describe the subject's behavior in rather direct ways, other CQ-items demand of the judge far-ranging inferences as to the subject's personality capabilities and latent motivational structure. Sometimes, judges express uneasiness about the extrapolations required of them.

The problem posed by highly inferential judgments is, of course, not one limited to the CQ-set. It is a problem generated by an acceptance of the conceptual necessity of employing "genotypical" or "metapsychological" variables for an understanding of personality. Contemporary orientations in psychiatry and personality psychology have chosen—and we support this conceptual choice—to employ abstract and directly unspecifiable constructs as means of making sense of behavior that seems otherwise bewilderingly diverse. Accordingly, the problem of inferential judgment must be lived with if we are to employ this conceptual orientation.

The process of clinical inference, of how an understanding develops by an accretion and integration of separately insufficient observations, cannot be discussed here.[20] The immediate practical dilemma about which we speak is what to do when a judge is required to describe a subject by means of the CQ-set but does not feel he has an adequate observational basis for inferring subject characteristics.

If the judge still has an opportunity to extend his observations of the little known subject, he should do so. When time must have a stop, however, the course of action is simply and bluntly for the judge to do the best he can. Using his implicit personality theory as an integrating guide, the judge should let the extrapolations from his scanty information go as they will. That is, he should sort the complete set of CQ-items.[21] He may be right, he may well be wrong. The important point to recognize is that if these conjectures do not issue with disproportionate frequency from certain judges, and if these conjectures are not preoccupied with certain classes of subjects, then the wildest of speculations will introduce no systematic bias. Discriminations will be more difficult to obtain and larger research samples will be needed than would otherwise be the case but no positive errors will be created. Moreover, if consensus descriptions are the research rule, then the importance of this source of error is greatly diminished.

Obviously, when a judge clearly has had no genuine opportunity to form an understanding of his subject, it would be ridiculous to force him to express a personality formulation. The result is likely to look like Everyman. In most research situations, however, judges will have had reasonably equivalent opportunities to assess subjects. In such circumstances, the confidence or absence of confidence of a judge in his evaluation of a subject's personality is no guide to the validity of the evaluation. This wry and to-be-respected fact derives now from a number of

---

[20] The reader will find it profitable to refer to a recent book devoted exclusively to this complex cognitive operation (Sarbin, Taft, & Bailey, 1960).

[21] Items should not be deleted from the CQ-set in order to make life easier for the judges. Such deletions would upset the comparability of the resulting data with data collected using the complete CQ-set. The more important reason for not considering the judges' comfort with inference is the distressing finding that different judges will wish deleted different Q-items. The implications of this situation are intolerable for the intent of the CQ-method would be defeated.

different studies (e.g., Forer & Tolman, 1952; Kelley & Fiske, 1951). An observer, while bewailing the insufficiencies of his information, may still be able to offer a most valuable evaluation of the subject.

Putting the point alternatively, a judge's satisfaction or concern with the information at his disposal may be viewed as a kind of "response set" (Cronbach, 1950). Some judges can never be satisfied that they know enough to evaluate a person; other observers are comfortable with grand extrapolations based upon flimsy data. To the extent that a judge's feeling that he has insufficient information is based upon a response characteristic of the judge, it is irrelevant to the presently defined purpose and should, sympathetically, be disregarded.

The problem involved in the use of the CQ-items, then, aside from matters of procedural detail, may be seen to be *not* specific to Q. These are large issues, issues that affect all efforts, however expressed, at the understanding of individuals and the communication of such understanding.

Chapter VI

THE METHODOLOGY OF Q-SORTING

In this chapter, we are concerned with three questions of Q-sort method which, over the years, have generated much discussion and some argument. Although to a great extent the problems to be considered are not unique to the Q-sort method but are problems of judgment generally, they require presentation again here. Only by an understanding of these issues can the Q-procedure as it responsively has evolved be in turn understood. The three questions we consider are:

1) Shall the Q-sorter fit his evaluations to a prescribed distribution or shall he be permitted a more spontaneous, more personal arrangement of O-items? This is the rather general issue of free versus forced-choice responses (Block, 1956).

2) If a forced distribution is decided upon, what form shall this distribution have?

3) In "characterizing" a personality, on what basis (and with what reliability) can a judge make use of and integrate Q-items which partake of so many different levels and facets of personality?

On employing a "forced" Q-distribution. The imposition of a standard or "forced" distribution of Q-items upon all Q-sorters has proven to be a controversial feature of the Q-sort method. Why should a judge of personality be forced to sort his items of description into a distribution he never made, into a suit of categories that may fit upon him in unnatural and uncomfortable ways?[22]

---

[22] To the writer, weary and abraded after long argument on this issue, it has sometimes seemed that opposition to the forcing feature of the Q-sort method has been based upon a peculiar connotative generalization or extension of word meanings. Psychologists and psychiatrists almost universally hold to an egalitarian, anti-

The logic underlying the forcing requirement in the Q-sort procedure needs to be understood for it aims to meet, in a reasonable way, a necessary requirement set by our defined goal of comparable descriptions. Perhaps the most convenient introduction to the rationale of the method is by way of illustrating the consequences when a prescribed distribution is *not* imposed.

Suppose in describing a subject, one judge evaluates many more items as extremely characteristic or extremely uncharacteristic than does the second judge, who is less assertive about his perceptions. In subsequently developing a consensus to serve as a better single formulation of the subject, the first judge by virtue solely of the extremeness of his response (and his larger variance) will tend to dominate the consensus judgment. There is enough evidence now (Valentine, 1929; Polansky, 1941; Kelley & Fiske, 1951; Forer & Tolman, 1952; Block, 1956) to suggest that assuredness of judgment is no promise of accuracy but is more often an undesirable response set. Accordingly, it is better to avoid this source of disproportionate weighting.

Consider now another kind of problem that arises from differences in the way judges segment a continuum. Let us suppose that two judges in characterizing a given personality *rank-order identically* the items of a Q-set. The items chosen as salient or defining of the subject by the one judge correspond exactly with the items selected by the second judge. In this most unlikely but paradigmatic situation the correlation *index* expressing agreement between the two judges is unity, and it would be said that perfect congruence in evaluation exists.

Now, suppose that these equivalent continua of items are to be recorded not as rank-orderings but as dichotomizations. The

---

authoritarian ethic. Consequently (i.e., given a connotative generalization), the idea *per se* of being *forced* and of *submitting* to this force is anathema, even if the context involved is as ego-irrelevant as the Q-sort procedure. A *free, unforced, spontaneous* arrangement of items somehow is more compatible with our needs for personal autonomy.

In this connection, I am reminded of the definition of *independent* and *dependent* variables offered by an apocryphal graduate student. "The *independent variable* is a *self-confident, self-reliant, personally autonomous, vigorous* kind of variable where the *dependent variable* is a *passive, trusting, indecisive,* and *immature* kind of dimension."

judges are separately asked to identify those items characteristic of the subject and those items not characteristic of the subject.

Now, the extent of the manifest agreement between judges will be strongly influenced by the way each of the judges chooses to dichotomize his continuum. For example, suppose one judge, with stringent standards as to what shall be called "characteristic" of a subject decides to sever the continuum so as to call only 10 items as characteristic (and 90 consequently as uncharacteristic). The second judge, however, more generously or more laxly partitions the items into a 90-10 split. This situation is illustrated in Table 6. Although from our definition of the situation we know the underlying order of the items to be identical, it can now be

TABLE 6

ILLUSTRATION OF THE EFFECTS ON AGREEMENT OF
RADICALLY DIFFERENT DICHOTOMIZATION

		Judge B		
		Character-istic of S	Uncharacter-istic of S	
	Characteristic of S	10	0	10
Judge A				
	Uncharacteristic of S	80	10	90
		90	10	

seen that the judges disagree on 80 of the 100 items, a most distressing situation. For all we know or are entitled to say now, Table 6 may even be describing a curvilinear relationship between the two judges. We know the underlying continua to be equivalent but are unable to assert the fact.

Only if both judges section the underlying continuum identically will the perfect correspondence be visible which we know to exist in this illustration. Conversely, *to the extent that judges differ among themselves in regard to their categorizing proclivities, their degree of manifest correlation will be unfairly attenuated.*

This last point is most important and, moreover, is not limited to the particular simple situation we have used to illustrate it. Where evaluations are expressed in more intervals than a dichotomy but in less detail than a complete rank-ordering, an essential agreement among judges may be obscured if judges distribute their Q-items in highly individual ways. As soon as the number of items exceeds the number of categories, the correspondence of different item arrangements becomes influenced by the *shapes* of the contrasted item distributions as well as by their orderings. The greater their divergence with regard to shape, with item ordering held constant, the more attenuated is the index of agreement between the two arrangements of items. Never, by the logic of the circumstance, can the index of correspondence between two observers be falsely elevated by unusual differences between the shape of item distributions.

Now, the intention of the Q-sort method in general and the CQ-set in particular is to assess the similarities and differences among Q-item orderings. Consequent upon the above logical finding that differences in the shape of item distributions upset the desired comparisons, it would follow as one alternative that every sorter should completely rank-order the Q-items with which he has to deal.

Unfortunately a complete rank-ordering of items is an unrealistic demand to make upon judges. The time required of the judge increases quite markedly for very many more discriminations are required. Moreover, the finer the discriminations demanded, the less the assuredness with which an item is placed —to the point where item ranks may show almost no stability at certain portions of the ranking spectrum.

For these several reasons—the excessive time required, the extreme personal difficulty with which a complete ranking is achieved by the judge, the fluctuations of items by several rank positions because of the unreliability of their placements—for these reasons, it proves not practical to accept complete rank-ordering as a solution of the problem posed by different "shapes" of item distributions.

Thus, we are forced to operate with a less-than-complete rank-ordering, i.e., to employ categories which are ordered relative to each other but within which further item discriminations are not made. With this necessity imposed, the obfuscation stemming from idiosyncratic item distributions is upon us once more. And now, the only remaining solution is to require that all judges place identical numbers of items into each of the prescribed categories—the "forced" sorting method. By employing a universal distribution for Q-items, comparisons become fair and straightforward for the arbitrarily-operating response sets of judges are prevented from arising. With highly variable, capriciously-determined distributions for items, comparisons are muddled and are just plain awkward to make.

The argument in favor of prescribing the distribution of items for the Q-sorter has thus far been a rationale one. But just as it is useful frequently to check one's algebra by a bit of arithmetic, it is useful too to test empirically the alternative consequences of the forced and unforced Q-sorting procedures. What we now describe in summary form is a study reported several years ago (Block, 1956) on exactly this issue. It merits mention that another study has more recently been completed at Minnesota which corroborates the essential conclusions of the earlier study.[23]

One of the persistent arguments against the employment of a prescribed Q-distribution has been that the forced-choice approach loses certain "information" which would be retained if an unforced distribution of judgments were tolerated. The suggestion here is that something important is being expressed about a subject when the judge describing him uses an unusual shape for the arrangement of items. It might be relevant indeed if one subject tended to elicit one kind of distribution from judges while another subject "pulled" a different distribution form.

Obviously, this point has merit and possibility. But it is an emphasis which properly should be brought into the empirical realm. It is not sufficient to assert simply that a methodological constraint loses "information." With the assertion devolves a responsibility to specify of what this "information" consists and just how important in the over-all scheme of things this information may be. There is information and there is "information," for not all of the reliable facets of behavior are worthy of consideration. Some are trivial or irrelevant to the predictive purpose at hand. Others are important but are reflected more completely or more directly by alternative means. *A priori*, the remark that the forced Q-sorting procedure excludes certain channels of

---

[23] Personal communication from P. E. Meehl.

communication should be interpreted not so much as a criticism but rather as a call for investigation of the weight and uniqueness of the eliminated information.

And so a study was designed to bear upon this question. Judges were asked to Q-sort a set of public people in a free and unrestrained way before the procrustean distribution was forced upon them. The design of the research was such as to permit assessment of the relative contributions of judges and of the observed subjects to the shape of the unforced distribution.

The primary and clear finding was that the judge idiosyncracies appeared to explain, almost completely, the various shapes of the unforced distributions of items. Judges differed among themselves radically and except in one instance which we mention immediately below, *not* as a function of the characteristics of the persons being described. An important ancillary finding is that in the unforced situation, judges did *not* volunteer certain discriminations they were able to make reliably when forced to the task.

Although the characteristics of the unforced distribution could be ascribed almost completely to judge idiosyncracies and not to the focus of interest, the subjects being evaluated, in one instance a subject did appear to influence systematically the unforced Q-item arrangements of the judges. The several sorters, when in the unforced situation, tended to employ the extreme scale categories significantly more often for this one subject than for the other people who were described.

This finding of course requires attention, for it is the kind that the forced situation precludes from existence. What then is the importance and psychological meaning of the observation that a particular subject "pulls" an especially extreme reaction from his judges?

Be it noted first that this characteristic of a subject simply exists with an unknown significance until it is related to other variables which can lend meaning to what otherwise remains simply an observation. In the study being cited, rather than embark upon a completely new experiment to discern the implications of this one subject-based determinant of the unforced Q-distribution, it proved convenient to analyze the *independent* data from the forced-sort situation. By comparing the forced item-orderings for the extremely viewed subject with the forced item-orderings for the other subjects, the uniquely large dispersion of the one subject stood revealed as due to his being perceived as *machiavellian, assertive, affectless, flamboyant,* and so on.

While there may be other implications of this individual's large dispersion that are not touched upon by the items included in the Q-set used in this study, the number and nature of the differtiating items make it seem likely that the central and derivative meanings of this subject's tendency to elicit extreme reactions were well expressed by the available Q-items. *If the reliable dispersion difference due to this subject's "pull" had beeen eliminated by the forcing procedure, it appears that little psychological information would have been lost,* for most of the meaning of this "pull" was already available from an examination of the Q-item *order.*

The instance described above is not an isolated finding. *In almost all Q-sort circumstances the psychological meaning of reliable distribution differences—both subject-based and judgebased—is also available or could be made available from examination of Q-item content.* The reason why this assertion is likely to be true is that for each of the recognized or conceivable variables which might create distribution differences in the unforced sorting situation, it is impossible to write a Q-item whose position in a forced sort would convey the meaning of the variable. Thereby, the need for a less direct and more equivocal measure of that variable via the unrestrained sorting procedure is eliminated.

Already noticed or hypothesized as creating distribution differences are such variables as "favorableness-unfavorableness" of evaluations, the amount of information the sorter feels is available to him, and the "colorfulness-drabness" of the object's personality. Variation with respect to each of these attributes can be expressed by the placement of suitable items within the forced sort. That is, if wide dispersion in the unforced sort reflects "colorfulness," then an item, "Is colorful," would by its placement within the forced sort convey the meaning of the eliminated dispersion measure. If the average scale value for items or the skewness of the unforced distribution are related to the "favorableness-unfavorableness" of the judge's evaluation, then items bearing upon favorable and unfavorable characteristics by their positioning in the forced sort will provide the same information as the eliminated elevation or skewness indices.

The only limitation on this stratgem for eliminating consideration of possible unforced distribution differences is that the Q-set being used in the constrained fashion must be comprehensive enough to include the various meanings of these "shape" differences. But this is only another way of saying that the Q-set must permit comprehensive personality description—a requirement we have already admitted and taken to heart.

On the relative merits of the freely evolved versus the prescribed distribution of Q-items, the following points summarize our several arguments and observations:

1) The unforced Q-sorting procedure obscures recognition of the correspondences existing among evaluations of personality where the forced Q-sorting procedure permits a clear assessment of degree of equivalence.

2) The unforced Q-sorting procedure tends to provide fewer discriminations than the forced Q-sorting procedure and consequently, is more susceptible to the Barnum effect (Meehl, 1956), the tendency to say very general and very generally true things about an individual.

3) The unforced Q-sorting procedure is not more reliable than is the forced Q-sorting procedure, even though with the latter procedure judges are required to make discriminations they otherwise are inclined not to offer.

4) The unforced Q-sorting procedure does not appear to provide information not also, and more easily, accessible through the forced Q-sorting procedure.

5) The unforced Q-sorting procedure provides data which is unwieldly and at times impossible to work with where the forced Q-sorting procedure provides data in a convenient and readily processed form.

For these multiple reasons, Stephenson's original requirement that each Q-sorter arrange his items in a fixed and specified distribution is reaffirmed here. The gains accruing from this device seem unquestionably to outweigh the costs of the imposition.[24]

On the form of the forced distribution. With the decision made to prescribe a Q-distribution, we must now concern ourselves with the question of just what distribution to fix upon.

In principle, it would be possible to find empirically the one best distribution for all judges to employ. Such a study, however, would be a complicated and arduous one if gone about in a sufficiently systematic manner so that a proper generalization would follow. Moreover, the question itself is not an especially decisive one.

There appear to be enough pertinent observations in the literature and arising out of Q-sort experience to permit by-passing a fully empirical approach to this less-than-crucial issue. As we shall see, various reasonings and findings all seem to converge upon a form for the distribution which it is unlikely a grand study on this issue could change significantly.

A first decision has to do with the symmetry-asymmetry of the decided-upon distribution. There would appear to be no formal reason for symmetry—all we require is that all sorters employ the same distribution, whatever be its form. But obviously a distribution to be used by many judges on many subjects should be as neutral or uncommitted as possible. Certainly a skewed distribution is too special a form to adopt. And so *the prescribed distribution should be symmetric.*

A second decision has to do with the number of categories to be employed along the judgmental continuum. Obviously, the more categories the better, for we have more discriminations. But use of too many categories might pressure the judge to the point where he responds with great difficulty and great randomness. *A distribution should have a fixed but sensible number of judgment categories.*

For a specific implementation of this assertion, there is abun-

---

[24] For those unpersuaded on this point but who may nevertheless be inclined to employ Q-sort technique, it is suggested that both unforced and forced Q-sortings be employed and studied. Following the unforced sort and recording of these data, the items can then be forced into the prescribed distribution. The additional labor is very slight and the alternative data-sets can then be interestingly compared.

dant pertinent information in the literature (Guilford, 1954, Ch. 11). From the many studies that have been done on rating methods, it is clear that judges can reliably discriminate up to 20 points on a rating scale. In our own practice, and after some trial and error, we have settled upon nine categories as sufficient and yet not too much. Other investigators have used alternate numbers of categories and Stephenson himself has used as many as 13. Our own experience indicates a nine interval continuum, although demanding of the judge, still elicits reliable discriminations. Admitedly, the choice might have gone either way—to increase or decrease the number of judgment categories by several. Nothing fundamental would be changed. The need for standardization is paramount here, however, if only for the convenience it affords and for that reason alone, the earlier decision to fix upon nine categories for the CQ-distribution continues to control present practice.

A third decision has to do with the essential shape of the symmetric distribution. By a misinterpretation of Stephenson, there has developed an understanding among many psychologists that a Q-distribution must be normal or Gaussian. This is not so, as Stephenson points out (1953, p. 60). The distribution may be of any non-bizarre shape, depending on the kinds of analyses proposed for the resulting data and depending too on just how congenial or affronting the judges expected to employ the prescribed distribution find it to be.

The reason for the widespread acceptance of the unnecessary and even inappropriate notion of a normal Q-distribution comes from a fundamental misunderstanding of the role and meaning of a correlation coefficient between Q-sorts. (See Chapter VII, below.)

The limiting possibilities for a symmetrical Q-distribution are a unimodal distribution, a rectangular or uniform distribution, and a U-shaped distribution. In a unimodal distribution, there is a piling up of items in the middle categories of the continuum; in a rectangular distribution, there are an equal number of items in each of the categories; in a U-shaped distribution, there is a predominance of items in the extreme categories with a de-emphasis of item placement in the middle categories. Of course, a distribution may be unimodal or U-shaped in varying degrees. Which of these distributions, or what amalgam of these alternatives, provides a reasonable distribution for all judges to employ?

We invoke at this point consideration of the number of discriminations afforded by a particular distribution shape. With the number of scale intervals or categories fixed, the number of discriminations in a Q-sort is solely a function of the shape of the distribution used.

The maximal number of discriminations comes from a rectangular distribution. To the extent that items pile up in any category, the total number of discriminations offered tends to decrease. Why not use, then, a rectangular distribution for Q-sorting in order to maximize discriminations?

This suggestion has in fact been made (Livson & Nichols, 1956) and it may be the one that should be followed. Our own reasoning has deferred somewhat—if not completely—to the "natural" distribution offered by judges in the unforced situation. In the free Q-sorting situation, the preferred distribution of items, averaged across a number of judges, appears to be a symmetric, somewhat unimodal one. It is definitely not normal in form, but instead verges toward rectangularity.

Besides this empirical observation, some introspective considerations and some statistical ones appear to converge upon equivalent solutions. For most Q-sorters, the extreme judgments are the easiest ones to offer; it is the discriminations in the middle portion of the continuum that are difficult and less reliable. At the same time, by the definition of the categories, middle placement of an item implies that it is relatively unimportant as a characteristic of the person being described.

Now, since mid-range discriminations do not contribute much information and also are most difficult to make, it would be helpful to sorters if precisely these discriminations were made fewer in number. We can accomplish this end simply by deviating from rectangularity toward unimodality.

From the statistical quarter, unimodality makes a kind of sense, too. One of the ways in which Q-data may be analyzed requires the use of an index of similarity between Q-sorters. Usually this similarity index is a correlation coefficient, an index which is especially sensitive to extreme item placement but which de-emphasizes the importance of items categorized close to the distribution's average. As long as such indices are used—and there is good reason for their use—it would seem wasteful of effort to gather finely-grained discriminations which will not be attended to by the indices we subsequently employ.

Although a rectangular Q-distribution provides the most discriminations, we have listed four reasons why *a Q-distribution should deviate somewhat away from rectangularity toward a unimodal distribution.* These are:

1) The one study which speaks to this issue (Livson & Nichols, 1956) has shown a somewhat unimodal distribution to be preferred, on the average, by a set of judges.

2) Items placed in middle categories are less important than extremely placed items in developing the psychological portrayal of the subject.

3) Items placed in the middle categories represent most difficult and time-consuming judgments for the sorter to make.

4) The conventional indices used to express the similarity between Q-sorts pay rather little attention to discriminations made in the mid-range.

For all of these reasons, an item-distribution was decided upon for the CQ-set which is unimodal but is flatter by far than a normal distribution. As can be seen from the number of items in each of the nine categories, 5, 8, 12, 16, 18, 16, 12, 8, 5, it is clearly not close to rectangularity either. However, in terms of the number of discriminations offered by this distribution (as computed by the method of Ferguson, 1949) it does not especially suffer in comparison with the number of discriminations offered by a nine-interval rectangular distribution. A rectangular distribution would provide 4400 discriminations where the CQ-distribution contributes 4349 discriminations. The numerical difference would not appear to be an important one, in the light of the reasons for deviating toward unimodality.

Obviously, from the relativistic nature of our arguments, the specific CQ-distribution adopted could have been somewhat different—either further toward or further away from rectangularity. But again, the standardization emphasis must be brought to bear in support of continued usage of the distribution as originally specified.

On "characterizing" a personality. In Appendix B is contained the instructions given to an evaluator to instruct and to guide him in his use of the method. For the initiate judge, these instructions provide a brief orientation to the procedure and its purpose, and suggest a convenient way of carrying out the task.

One of the concerns expressed by Q-sorters has to do with the nature of the dimension along which items are to be ordered. How is this dimension to be understood? On what basis are Q-items which are obviously diverse or even at different levels of analysis to be compared against each other and scaled along the same continuum? How can a phenotypical Q-item like "Initiates humor" be contrasted with a more inferential item such as "Has a readiness to feel guilty?" Surely, it has been suggested, the item comparisons required in Q-sorting are the comparisons of apples with oranges, of things sensibly non-comparable. The ordering of items so as to describe an individual is, from this point of view, simply not a meaningful task.

The preceding concern is in many ways an understandable one. Certainly the Q-sorter very frequently experiences doubt, indecision, and despair over the actions required of him. The wondrous and well-established fact, however, is that the behavior of the Q-sorter is highly repeatable (test-retest reliabilities of .8 and .9 are conventional).[25] Frank (1956) in a small study reports Q-sort test-retest reliabilities ranging from .93 to .97! Despite his personal sense of uncertainty, the consistency with which a sorter can evaluate Q-items along an abstract and complex dimension is a very striking finding. And the establishment of high reliability for a Q-sort of course implies that something meaningful is captured by the item-ordering. Whether that

---

[25] The judge's specific memory for how he placed Q-items in his first sorting is not an important factor falsely elevating these reliabilities. The number of Q-items far exceeds the capacity of memory. Moreover, retroactive inhibition by intervening Q-sortings of other subjects also operates to destroy memory of the precise arrangement of items in the first sorting. The consistency over time appears instead to be due to the equivalent expression on separate occasions of an unchanged conception of the subject.

meaningful something is the underlying dimension we desire is another question which we must consider. For the present we wish to emphasize that ipsative ratings can be offered as reliably as are normative ratings.

The questioning by psychologists of ipsative ratings together with their simultaneous acceptance of normative ratings can be seen as based on the tradition and familiarity surrounding the latter description technique, not on its intrinsic superiority. It is not more "natural" to rate a group of subjects on the variable of "impulsivity," partialling out the social and personality context in which the impulsivity should be understood, than it is to evaluate the function of "impulsivity" in an individual's personality without regard to how that individual stands on the dimension in relation to other members of a group. Both approaches require an abstraction out of context. Historically we just happen to have employed the one artifice more often than the other; hence the sense of security with which normative ratings are offered. The ability of judges to use both rating orientations with high personal reliabilities is operational evidence for a meaning in each. The question of relative usefulness will of course depend upon the particular experimental context at hand.

We go on now to discuss the proper nature of the complex dimension along which items are to be ordered. What is the criterion which must be served by the sorter?

It is suggested that the criterion to be used to guide the Q-sorter in his difficult task should be informational in nature. By informational here, reference is to the sense in which the concept of information is employed in information theory (e.g., Attneave, 1959) and in measurement logic (Cronbach, 1953).

The goal is to characterize a personality by means of the available Q-items. The sorter selects items in terms of their "intrapersonal salience," placing positively "salient" items toward one end of the continuum and negatively "salient" items toward the other end. Items which are not salient fall into middle categories. What then shall we mean by the notion of "salience"? Here the informational criterion provides a definition.

Of two Q-items, the item *excluding* the most behavioral

alternatives (or believed by the judge to do so) is by definition most "salient." An item is "not salient" if it fails to delimit in any way the range of behaviors or characteristics of the person being described.

The limiting cases, according to this definition, are where an item permits or predicts only one behavioral possibility (and is therefore most "salient") and where an item does not at all limit the set of behavior alternatives (and is therefore irrelevant to the personality formulation). Some examples may help to convey the meaning of this criterion definition. But first, let us attempt a justification of this definition of salience. For many, the notion of predicting what it is an individual will *not* do seems "unnatural" and so, a few statements of the rationale here are in order.

This "unnatural" definition is favored here over the more conventional aim to predict specifically for two reasons.

1) It is in general impossible to offer seriously highly specific predictions in psychology. This is not to deny pin-pointed prediction as the ultimate aspiration of the science; it is simply to recognize the complexities we wish to specify and the poor tools at our command. Moreover, in the isolated instances where pin-pointed prediction is feasible, it is but a limiting case of the alternative definition favored here.

2) Pin-pointed predictions leads to a confusion and neglect with regard to the predictions that are "good misses" since a specific prediction is either "right" or "wrong." To predict that an individual, because of anxiety, is going to be subject to a radical reorganization of his personality is a delimiting type of prediction. To predict that this individual, as a function of his anxiety level, will cheat on a particular examination is a pin-pointed prediction. To test only highly specific predictions is proving for the present a premature effort. But we can test our knowledge of personality functioning if we choose to operate at a more general level. We require an infinite amount of information to say what someone is but can begin with much less information to say what someone is not. The latter approach of excluding alternatives is more humble but allows us signs of

progress toward the ultimate and limiting case of eliminating all alternatives but one.

As an illustration of the preceding point of view, consider a game wherein a person is to be described by one and only one statement. Perhaps a college youth is wiring home a ten-word message—all he can afford to send—informing his parents for the first time of his impending marriage and requesting some emergency funds. If the funds are to be sent by his parents, it is necessary that they know what sort of person their son is marrying. Being aware of this intolerance of ambiguity on the part of his parents, just how should the enterprising youth compose his telegram? What one descriptive statement of 10 words would provide most information to the receivers of the message?

He could write "Getting married to member of human race. Send money. Love." Or even, "Getting married to a girl. Send money. Love, love, love." On the assumption that the groom's psychosexual development has been reasonably normal, neither of these messages would give his parents any clue at all as to the sort of person their son is marrying. In our present terms, these messages would not be conveying salient features of the bride's personality.

A better message—better in the sense that closer specification of the nature of the girl is posible—might be, "Getting married to sociology graduate student. Send money. Love, love." Certainly, female sociology graduate students are a more homogeneous group than girls in general, and accordingly, this message should leave the boy's parents rather more informed. By our conventions, the message has eliminated some behavioral alternatives and the information provided is therefore salient.

An even more informative telegram might be, "Getting married to acutely disturbed hebephrenic schizophrenic. Send money. Love." The message—distressing as it would be—is extremely specifying of the girl's characteristics. As a group, female acutely disturbed schizophrenics are more homogeneous characteristically than female graduate students in sociology. Such a descriptive statement, if it applied, would be an extremely salient one.

By further refining the description of a person, his character is delineated ever more closely. That is, having classified a person

—and the classification may be based upon many variables—we have, if the classifying variables are behaviorally relevant, eliminated many behaviors as possibly emanating from that person.

Now as we play the game, we are not at a telegraph office chewing a pencil and pondering over the poor quality of parental understanding. We have, in the CQ-set, 100 possible messages to "send." Judgments of salience are thus strictly limited by the particular items made available. Items that are not included in the specified ensemble—be they too universal in nature ("is a member of the human race") or too molecular ("has a reaction time of .12 second to a supra-threshold electric shock") or merely unfortunate omissions—are irrelevant to the immediate problem before the judge of personality, namely, sorting the particular set of cards he has been given. Because judgments and comparisons can be made only between those items included in the Q-deck, in order to avoid *post-hoc* regrets here is another reason for exhaustive coverage by an item-set.

The Q-sorter is in the position of having to decide from among the 100 items in the CQ-set, which set of 10 statements (five positively phrased items and five negatively phrased items) he judges as most informative, as defining most decisively the personality of the person being described. Having selected this set of most salient items, he then considers anew the remaining 90 items and selects the set of 16 statements (eight positive and eight negative items) which, of the 90, are now the most salient items. And so on, to the completion of categorization.

A final complicating remark on salience and what may be called "meta-salience." Many Q-items may be critically informative for the simple reason that they are judged *not* salient for this particular subject—these items are "meta-salient." For example, if an item like "Has high aspiration level for self" is sorted into a middle category in describing a subject, information still has been conveyed. This person is viewed as not dominated or driven by ambition, nor yet as a passive, defeated individual. By the item's placement, the judge is expressing his evaluation that for this subject aspirations and problems having to do with aspirations do not provide a central theme in terms of which the personality is to be understood. Certainly this is important information. Its importance, however, derives from a different context of understanding that the salience context in which judgments are initially offered.

This, then, is how the dimension of "salience" along which the Q-items are to be placed takes on its meaning. A personality is portrayed by the items the judge evaluates as important, characteristic, or defining of the person being described. In practice, the foregoing rationale operates only implicitly and judgments proceed apace. For this reason, it is important every so often to call attention to the meaning of the sorting continuum, if only to re-sensitize the judges to the purpose of their task.

Chapter VII

RESEARCH APPLICATIONS OF THE CQ-SET

By this point of the present monograph, a diligent reader should be in a position to carry out and to record a Q-sort, even if not on a routine basis. The procedure, however, is not designed simply to provide data in a special format. We must turn now to a discussion of the purposes to which these standard-form evaluations can be put. In what kinds of research are these data likely to prove useful?

Some illustrations of CQ-set applications were offered in the first chapter. It would appear that the various analytical possibilities of the CQ-procedure fall into essentially two categories, namely, analysis at the level of item-by-item comparisons and analysis, in a more total way, of the correspondence or similarity between Q-sorts. Within each of these broad classes, a pair of sub-classes may be elaborated. We propose to discuss the general methods of analysis of Q-data, indicating the scope of each type of application and spelling out where need be the technical operations that may prove useful. Some cautions and constraints are also noted where appropriate.

In the treatment of Q-sort data, the quantitative analysis of individual items has been relatively neglected, although where employed the approach has proven quite productive. Two kinds of item analysis of Q-data will be discussed here:

1) The comparison of item placements in one Q-sort with item placements in another Q-sort.

2) The comparison of Q-item placements in one group of individuals with Q-item placements in another group of individuals.

Q-data have most frequently been used in a "global" manner, where the *correlations or similarities among Q-sorts* are the basic data for analysis. These correlations among CQ-sorts are amenable to various interesting forms of treatment but also, unfortunately, to certain forms of misinterpretation. It is most important in these very useful comparisons of configurations that improper models for inference from these data be avoided.[26]

The similarities among CQ-sorts may be employed in two ways which are discussed under the headings:

1) The correspondence of Q-sorts with a criterion (or conceptual or defining) Q-sort.

2) The intercorrelation of Q-sorts to permit, via factor or cluster analysis (Hotelling, 1933; Thurstone, 1947; Tryon, 1958), the discernment of types or clusters of people.

COMPARING ITEM PLACEMENTS IN ONE Q-SORT WITH ITEM PLACEMENTS IN ANOTHER Q-SORT

Perhaps the most obvious usage of Q-evaluations is simply to contrast a pair of Q-descriptions in order to observe the items placed discrepantly in the two orderings. Two Q-sorting clinicians may wish to compare their impressions of the same patient; two psychologists interested in the study of creativity may wish to Q-sort their hypothetical conceptions of the creative individual in order to gain, from their item differences, recognition of their theoretical divergencies; and so on.

In order to know whether an item in one Q-ordering is placed differently in a second Q-arrangement, it is necessary to have some idea as to what difference in item placement is to be considered significant. If one sorter places an item at position 3 while a second sorter places the same item at position 4, is this a difference worth attending to, or does the difference between placements of an item have to be two intervals, or three intervals, or how many?

One can operate here with an informal criterion or with a

---

[26] Because of the special emphasis of the CQ-set, the presentation here is restricted to those methods of correspondence analysis that are relevant to *observer-evaluations*. Accordingly, certain procedures involving the correlation of *self-descriptive Q-data* are not discussed, although many of the general remarks to be made here will apply as well to self-sort data.

formal criterion as to what differences are to be considered significant. For most purposes, the informal way will identify adequately enough the items differentiating between the sorts and without the assumptions and labors the formal, i.e., statistical, method entails. The informal method suggested here is simply to line up the two Q-sorts to be compared and then to note the items where the two sortings differ by *three* or more intervals. After arranging these differentiating items by their direction of difference and by the magnitude of placement difference, a reading of these items portrays directly the nature of the differences between the two evaluations. In most circumstances where CQ-sorts are to be compared item by item, this decision method for selecting the differentiating items is precise enough.

For certain applications, however, a statistical basis for decision may be desired. The researcher may wish to know whether a discrepancy in item placement is, from a statistical point of view, a significant one. Given some conventional, but still disputed assumptions, psychometrics permits an answer to this question.

It is necessary first to have some idea of the chance variation to be expected for each item's placement, i.e., we need to know the standard error of the value or score assigned to each item. This standard error is a function of the reliability of the Q-sort and of the standard deviation of the Q-description. Specifically, the standard error of item placement σ_{ip}, is:

$$\sigma_{ip} = \sigma_D \sqrt{1 - \text{reliability of the } Q\text{-sort}} \quad (3)$$

where σ_D is the standard deviation of the Q-distribution. For the CQ-set, this σ_D is 2.08. With the typical reliabilities of .8 or .9 which are found with the CQ- set, the standard error of item placement is in the range from .91 to .66 of an interval.[27]

---

[27] The specific assumptions underlying this formula are (a) that the σ_{ip} is the same for all items and (b) that the σ_{ip} is the same along all parts of the nine-point sorting continuum. Both of these assumptions are known not to be correct in any strict sense of the word. Since the reliabilities of individual Q-items differ somewhat among themselves, individual σ_{ip}'s ideally should be computed for each item. Also, it is well known that σ_{ip} is smaller for items placed at extreme scale positions than it is for items placed in middle positions. Accordingly, a more rigorous formula which recognizes the degree of extremeness of an item's placement (McHugh, 1957) would provide more appropriate results.

By applying formula (3), an *average* σ_{ip} is derived which when applied to par-

We now need to calculate the standard error of the *difference* between the values assigned by the two sorters to the item under scrutiny. This standard error of the difference depends on the separate standard errors of the Q-values. The required formula here is:

$$SE_{dip} = \sqrt{\sigma_{ip_1}^2 + \sigma_{ip_2}^2} \qquad (4)$$

where SE_{dip} is the standard error of the difference between the two Q-values, σ_{ip_1} is the standard error of item placement for the first sorter, and σ_{ip_2} is the standard error of item placement for the second sorter. In order to specify how large a discrepancy between item placements must be in order for it to be statistically significant at or beyond the conventional .05 or .01 levels, we simply multiply the SE_{dip} by 1.98 or 2.63, respectively.[28]

An illustration may clarify the foregoing. Let us suppose two CQ-sorts, one with a reliability of .85 and the other with a reliability of .81 are to be compared. How large a difference between Q-values is required in order for a discrepancy in item positions to be significant at the .05 level?

From formula (3), we compute the standard error of Q-values to be .81 for the first sorter and .91 for the second judge. Plugging these values (squared) into formula (4), we solve the expression and find the SE_{dip} in these instance to be 1.22 of an interval. We now multiply this SE_{dip} by 1.96, the .05 level multiplier, and find a difference of 2.39 intervals is significant at our specified level.

It should be recognized, however, that differences in the placement of O-items can take on *integer* values only. That is, since Q-scores can take on only nine *integer* values, differences in item placement also will be integers. Consequently, a difference of 2.39 intervals cannot be employed as a practical criterion

---

ticular Q-items may be in error to the extent the underlying assumptions are violated. However, the error is likely to be slight for the reliabilities of CQ-items, although different, do not appear to vary drastically, nor does the correction for extreme placement appreciably affect the σ_{ip} of a Q-item. In addition, it should be noted that later, when this σ_{ip} is used to develop an estimate of the difference in item placement required for statistical significance, a conservative factor is introduced which operates against the finding of *false* differences. All in all, therefore, this conventional means of estimating σ_{ip} would appear to be suitable for the present application.

[28] For exploratory research, it may be desirable to use as relaxed a requirement as significance at the .10 level. In this case, the multiplier for the SE_{dip} is 1.66.

of significance. We must move *up* to the closest integer, in this instance, the number *three,* and use this value as the criterion of significance. By using the next higher integer, a more stringent criterion of significance is being applied—a move toward conservatism in the results obtained. In the illustration above, then, differences in item placement of three or more intervals are significant beyond the .05 level.

Having presented a logic by which the significance of item differences may be statistically evaluated, a kind of justification can now be offered for the rough-and-ready method proposed earlier for identifying relevant discrepancies in item placement. From formulas (3) and (4), it can be seen that the size of the difference that will be significant is a function of the reliability of the Q-sorts and the level of significance set by the investigator. Now, for the range of reliabilities usually encountered and for the levels of significance conventionally set, a difference between Q-values of three intervals or more will almost invariably be significant beyond the .05 level.[29] Indeed, a difference of two intervals will quite frequently prove to be significant. Consequently, the quick and approximate method we have suggested works well and errs, if at all, on the side of conservatism. The highlights of the differences between sorts are detected; some actually significant differences in item placement may not be discerned.

As indicated earlier, only occasionally will a statistical basis for inferring the importance of differences in item placement be desired. The available statistical model for inference in this context is a parametric one, involving some reasonable assump-

---

[29] By way of illustration here, we may use an example where the finding of significant differences in item placement will tend to be minimized. When reliabilities are low, the size of the interval required for significance will increase. As the level of significance set by the investigator is made more stringent, the size of the interval required for significance will increase. Now, with reliabilities of .80—on the low side—at the .05 level a difference in item placement of 2.53 intervals is significant. A difference of 3.32 intervals is significant at the .01 level. Most often, investigators will be working with data of higher reliability. Accordingly, the criterion of a three interval difference or more may be seen to be a rapidly applied and conservative one. For inspectional purposes, differences of only two intervals are often considered.

tions that are usually but perhaps not always empirically approximated. Unless the special kind of support available from a statistical basis of inference is required, the more casual but still informative method of simply identifying the discrepantly placed Q-items is recommended. When the investigator does choose to employ the statistical approach, he should check carefully to see whether, in the data he will be evaluating, the assumptions of the model are approximated reasonably closely.

COMPARISON OF Q-ITEM PLACEMENTS IN ONE GROUP OF INDIVIDUALS

A rather frequent potential use of Q-data involves comparison, item by item, of the Q-sorts for one group of individuals and the Q-sorts for another group of subjects. In assessment situations, for example, an experimental procedure may group individuals who are autonomically reactive and individuals who are autonomically unreactive (Block, 1957c). Comparison of the Q-sorts for the individuals in the one group with the Q-sorts of the individuals in the other group—data that are completely independent of the basis of classification—can reveal the personality characteristics associated with autonomic hyper- and hyporeactivity. Or, in a psychiatric clinic, it may be possible to identify a group of patients who although scoring high on the Psychasthenia (Pt) Scale of the MMPI, score low on the Schizophrenia (Sc) Scale. As a rule, the correlation between these two scales is highly positive. Consequently, it would be of interest to study the nature of the patients in whom the usual relationship between Pt and Sc fails to obtain. If Q-sorts on patients are available, then the patients in whom the unusual Pt-Sc relationship exists can be contrasted with patients in whom the conventional patterning is found. An item by item comparison of the Q-sorts for each group would provide some light on the personality homogeneities and personality differences in and between the groups, as independently viewed by clinicians.

The essential requirement for comparison of the Q-sorts of one group with the Q-sorts of another group is that the basis for establishing the groups be independent of the Q-item placements.

We can compare "good" and "mediocre" officers, chess-players and dice-throwers, cheerleaders and accountants, psychotherapists and neurologists, the children of elderly parents and the children of young parents—the possible comparisons require only some imagination, an objective basis for identifying or classifying individuals and, of course, proper Q-sort data.

The specific procedures for Q-item analysis are simple, if tedious. For a given item, the distribution of Q-values or scores for the individuals in the first group is compared with the distribution which exists in the second group. If the one distribution, by statistical test, proves to be higher or lower than the other, then that item distinguishes the two groups. For example, for item j the scale values for individuals in one group may be 3, 4, 3, 5, 2, 3, 2, 4, 7, and 4. The scale values for this same item for individuals in a second group may be 6, 5, 7, 6, 6, 5, 9, 8, 6, and 7. Clearly, by inspection and also by statistics, the second distribution has a higher average than the first and accordingly we would say that item j is *more* characteristic in general of individuals in the second group.

In evaluating the significance of difference between the mean placements of a Q-item in two groups, the statistical test to be used depends on the nature of the distributions of Q-values. If the Q-values or scores for an item have a distribution which comports well enough with the requirements of parametric tests, then these may be used. When clearly the distribution of Q-values for a given item does not meet the assumptions underlying a parametric model or when the issue is in doubt, then distribution-free (i.e., non-parametric) tests should be employed.

Specifically, when two groups are being compared and the distributions of Q-values for a given item are reasonably symmetrical and have variances which are not too divergent, then Student's t test is perhaps the test of choice. When more than two groups are being evaluated with respect to a Q-item and the parametric assumptions are tenable, then the F test is appropriate. These tests are described in almost any elementary statistical text, e.g., McNemar (1955). When parametric assumptions are to be avoided, then the most efficient two-sample test to discern differences in Q-item placement is the Mann-Whitney test (Mann

& Whitney, 1947). The extension of the Mann-Whitney test, for
the case where more than two groups are involved, is the *H* test
of Kruskal and Wallis (1952). A convenient secondary source
for both of these distribution-free tests is the volume by Walker
and Lev (1953). All of these tests are straightforward.

For each Q-item, the test of differences in item placement between the groups being compared must be done. Different
Q-items will have different dispersions (variances) within a group
of subjects and so an average standard error is clearly inappropriate. For the 100-item CQ-set, 100 significance tests are
required, an onerous task indeed If the work is to be performed
manually, then a systematization of the computational procedure
will both speed the effort and lessen the liklihood of error. The
investigator should be alerted to the increasing availability of
high-speed computers, a resource which makes computations
exceedingly inexpensive. With costs low and convenience at
hand, extensive data analyses which could not have been realized
previously can now be undertaken even on an exploratory basis.
From the results of the Q-data analyses of this kind that have
been done thus far, this general method promises to be a most
productive one.[30]

Several measurement and statistical considerations must now
be discussed, in order to clarify and justify certain features of this
general procedure. In the comparison of groups with respect
to their item placements, it should be noted that we are here
treating as normative, data which originally were collected
ipsatively (cf. Chapter 2). Initially, item *j* for individual *i* was
evaluated *vis-a-vis* the remaining 99 items being used to characterize individual *i*, and in this context it was assigned to a
category, i.e., given a scale value. Now, we are taking individual

---

[30] It must be noted that occasionally, investigators have employed the procedure of
contrasting average Q-sorts for each group, noting item placement divergencies ex-
ceeding a pre-set amount. This method is a faulty one, even when statistical
considerations are invoked in determining the size of the discrepancy to be treated
as significant. The reason is that in any application of a Q-set, different Q-items will
have different dispersions. Statistical comparisons, item-by-item, respect these variance differences; the application of a standard criterion of difference, by neglecting
this factor, commits mistakes which may well be important.

i's value for item *j* and comparing it with the ipsatively earned values for item *j* of *other* individuals. This is now normative measurement and some concern has been expressed as to the appropriateness of this usage (Cattell, 1944, p. 296; Guilford, 1954, p. 528).

This methodological concern is accessible to empirical study and elsewhere, a test of the propriety of employing ipsatively-collected data as normative scores has been reported (Block, 1957a). It may be said, as a result of this study, that the normative treatment of ipsative scores such as proposed here is well justified empirically. The kinds of discriminations afforded by normative data treated normatively and by ipsative data treated normatively appear to be fully equivalent and functionally interchangeable, at least in the one direction where we ask ipsative data to "act" like normative scores.

Another problem develops from the fact that Q-values are not completely independent of each other, a situation which may complicate the interpretations to be drawn from the set of 100 significance tests, when each of the CQ-items is analyzed. There are two ways in which lack of independence of values in a Q-sort is created. The first of these is a purely logical one, which proves to be unimportant in its effects in this context. The second cause of relation among Q-items is a substantive one, one which can be quite subtle in its ramifications and decisive in its consequences.

The logical basis for an interdependence among items stems from the employment of a forced distribution of Q-values. By the placing of an item into a category, the likelihood is lessened that other items also will be placed in that category. This point is most readily seen by example. By the definition of the Q-distribution, only five items are permissibly assigned to category nine. After five items—any five items—have been so assigned, it follows that *none* of the 95 remaining items can have Q-values of 9. It is in this sense that we have a lack of independence of item placement. Items in one category displace other items from that category. This inter-dependence is of a *reciprocal* kind, for an item placed in an extreme position forces other items to be less extreme; an item placed in the middle of the continuum in effect forces other items to be extremely positioned. Thus, if a Q-item for each of the members of a group is placed at an extreme position while for the members of a second group, the item is not extremely placed, that item properly may prove to be a significant differentiator. But—and here the impact of the lack of independence is to be seen—because this one item was a significant differentiator, other items are less likely to be extremely placed and hence emerge as significant. The slightly negative correlation among Q-items imposed by the forced nature of the Q-distribution creates this effect.

The important question here, of course, is how potent is this disturbing influence? If the forced nature of the Q-distribution constrained item analyses from manifesting differences that in fact were present, then some adjustment of the total technique would be required. The answer, however, is that the negative correlation among items that is built in by the forcing feature of the method is most minute. If the number of Q-items was very small, the reciprocal effect could be important indeed. But as the number of items increases, and consequently the degrees of freedom available to the sorter, the forced negative correlation among items decreases almost to the vanishing point and indeed can be computed to be no greater than -.01 for a 100 item Q-set (Haggard, 1958, pp. 17-18). We can, therefore, neglect this most slight bias in our significance tests.

The second kind of interdependence among Q-items is a more important and even ubiquitous one which comes about from the operation of factors beyond the Q-sort method. It is well recognized that, in the nature of things, psychological variables will correlate. In general (but not without exception) *dominance* will correlate with *assurance, empathy* with *warmth*, and so on. And since Q-items are indices of underlying variables, they too will correlate with each other. Consequently, if a statistical test of one item's differentiating capacity proves to be significant, then the statistical tests of all the items correlated with the first item may be expected to have some tendency to be significant. The converse applies here too for if an item is *not* a differentiator, then all the items associated with this first item also will tend not to be differentiating.

Now, in the analysis of CQ-items, 100 significance tests are calculated. If all of these tests were independent of each other, then from classical statistical reasoning we would expect, for example, an average of 5% of them to be significant beyond the .05 level. In evaluating a *set* of 100 independent significant tests, we would insist that *reliably more* than 5% of the tests be significant. Otherwise, we would have no basis for believing the set of results to be based on anything other than chance.

But the multiple significance tests of the CQ-items are *not* independent of each other. The results of one item analysis do have implications for the results of other item analyses. How then can we form from these numerous separate significance tests, a proper evaluation of the full set of results? When shall we know that our findings are not most parsimoniously ascribed to the workings of chance? It should be emphasized that this kind of problem occurs rather often in psychological and other research where many measures are employed and analyzed. It is *not* a problem peculiar to the Q-sort method.

Until recently, there has been no means, other than the often unfeasible method of cross-validation, to deal with this question for conventional statistical models could not provide an appropriate basis of inference. Recently, an unbiased, empirical method for deciding whether a set of findings *qua* set is significant or not has been evolved (Block, 1960). The reader is referred to this paper for an extended discussion of the problem and the logic of the proposed solution. In brief, it may be said here that a computer is employed to generate empirically a sampling distribution of the number of significant differences to be expected on the basis of chance, when the originally obtained variance-covariance matrix of variables (Q-items) is used to delimit the population of possible sets of findings. The method is completely general and its results can be made as precise as desired simply by extending the time the computer operates.

In practice, then, the investigator will want to resort to the use of a computer in order not only to lessen the burdens of the Q-item analyses but also to permit a clear and unequivocal statement in regard to the significance of the full set of results. Where a computer is not accessible to an investigator, and where a specific hypothesis is not under test, analyses of Q-items will have to be cross-validated or be interpreted only provisionally.

THE CORRESPONDENCE OF Q-SORTS WITH A CRITERION (OR CONCEPTUAL OR DEFINING) Q-SORT

For certain forms of research questions, we may wish to know whether individuals in one group correlate more with a criterion than do individuals in a second group. For example, are the mothers of schizophrenic children more like the theoretical conception of the schizophrenogenic mother than are mothers of neurotic children? (Block, J. H., Patterson, Block, J., & Jackson, 1958); are clinicians more accurate in their inferences from a Rorschach than they are when inferring from the MMPI or CPI? (Shapiro, 1957); does the interpersonal situation of an individual determine the accuracy of his social perception? (Block & Bennett, 1955), and so on. In all of these instances, the emphasis is on over-all comparison of Q-sorts rather than the comparison of item placements.

Before discussing this analytical procedure, it is necessary first to discuss more generally some problems involved in assessing similarity between people. A first question, of course, is similarity with respect to what? In the present context, the 100 items in the CQ-set define the facets in terms of which and only in terms of which similarity and difference are to be understood. Again, the point is made that to the extent the CQ-set is inadequate, the notion of the similarity of two individuals described by means of the set loses meaning. Time and again, the comprehensiveness of the Q-set is seen to be a fundamental requirement.

But if we do choose to employ the CQ-set, how best is similarity to be indexed? With regard to this question, there has been a fair bit of controversy. Initially, Stephenson suggested that a product-moment correlation coefficient is quite sufficient, and this suggestion has been adopted in the large majority of Q-studies which have been reported. In 1953, an influential article by Cronbach and Gleser (1953) appeared which criticized the use of r as an index of similarity on the grounds that in certain research contexts, a correlational index of similarity neglects some important kinds of information. The alternative index which they proposed at the time, the D measure, has since seen some use in Q-sort and other contexts.

In the meanwhile, a greater perspective has been gained with regard to the specific circumstances wherein a simple correlation coefficient may fail to discriminate important qualities and those circumstances where it is a quite appropriate index of similarity. The decisive matter here is whether or not information is conveyed by the nature of the *unforced* distribution of Q-items. Where a forced Q-distribution is employed, the distinction between r and D vanishes for all the available information now duly affects the correlation coefficient.

As indicated in Chapter VI, the unforced distribution does not in the context of observer-evaluations of personality appear to provide unique kinds of information and so, when the forced distribution is employed, a correlation coefficient properly may be employed to index the extent of correspondence between two orderings of Q-items.

When it is desired to estimate the correspondence between two Q-sorts, a product-moment correlation coefficient is readily computed from the formula:

$$r = 1 - \frac{\sum d_{ip}^2}{2N\sigma_D^2} \qquad (5)$$

where d_{ip}^2 is the squared difference between the Q-values of corresponding items, N is the number of items in the Q-set and σ_D is the standard deviation of the Q-set. This well-known formula simplifies but is algebraically identical with the conventional formula for the correlation coefficient (cf., e.g., Cohen, 1957). For the CQ-set, with 100 items and a σ of 2.08, formula (5) simplifies to:

$$r = 1 - \frac{\sum d_{ip}^2}{864}$$

With a hand calculator, a correlation between two Q-sorts is rapidly computed for the only variable in the equation is the sum of *squared* discrepancies, all other quantities being constant. The largest possible discrepancy is 8 (the differences between a

Q-value of 9 for an item in one sort and a value of 1 for that item in the second sort). All the squares of discrepancies can be held in mind easily and the computation can proceed with great ease. This index may be computed by a deft calculator in less than two minutes. A table, applicable to the CQ-set, which permits reading the value of r when given $\sum d_{ip}^2$ is to be found in Appendix G.

It should be noted that the Q-sorting procedure is essentially a rank-order technique, where many ties are permitted. Strictly, an index of correspondence between rank-orders, such as Kendall's *tau*, would appear to be most appropriate to use for it does not make the assumption of an equal-interval scale which a correlation coefficient requires. The correlation coefficient continues to be suggested for use here, despite its stronger assumption, for several reasons. It is more readily computed; descriptively, it has a context of meaning which Kendall's *tau* and other rank-order indices do not yet enjoy; and—most important— the ordering of relationships among Q-sorts as indexed by the correlation coefficient essentially is equivalent to the ordering of relationships as revealed by a rank-order index. This latter property of r follows because r, except in bizarre or contrived instances, is a monotonic transformation of *tau*.

Several features of the correlation coefficient as an index of correspondence require elaboration before going on to its applications. Discrepancies in item placement are *squared* (for this is a product-moment index). The squaring procedure places an emphasis on large differences and gives much less weight to small discrepancies. By and large, this kind of emphasis is usually either desirable or at least not wrong for the kinds of application a similarity index will have. We tend to be interested, in psychology, more in differences than in similarity, and the index r accords with that preoccupation. Where such an emphasis is deemed undesirable, alternative indices may be constructed, as for example, the simple sum of discrepancies, which cuts down appreciably the role played by large differences.

By virtue of its status as a correlation coefficient, r as an index of the similarity of two Q-sorts has an intrinsic descriptive meaning. An r of .75 testifies to a very appreciable agreement between two sorts; an *r* of .15 signifies rather little correspondence—all of this following from our knowledge of the metrical properties of *r*. But, and here is the point of importance, in statistically evaluating the index *r*, we are *not* except in most unusual instances entitled to take advantage of the sampling distribution of the correlation coefficient as a basis for inference. The index *r* is for purposes of statistical inference essentially but a *score* and may be treated only by statistical techniques that respect the properties of that score and its particular obtained distribution. If we wish to know whether two Q-sorts are reliably similar, we cannot employ the conventional standard error formula for the correlation coefficient to test whether the index *r* is significantly different from zero. We must instead find a way to set the confidence limits for the score *r* from knowledge of the distribution of *r* in the sample of similarity scores with which we are working. If we wish to know whether two *r's* are significantly different, we cannot employ the usual formula for assessing the difference between two correlations; we must instead find the standard error of each of the *r* scores and estimate the importance of the difference by a *t*-test. Often, it may be difficult to find or to develop the desired standard errors, but proper planning and research design can usually permit the desired comparisons to be made. The important recognition to be had here is that no improper statistical inferences will be made if *r*, the index of similarity, is treated solely as a score and not as a correlation coefficient.

The basis for the foregoing assertions is not widely recognized and consequently, a fair number of errors of inference have been committed in the analysis of Q-correlations. The fundamental reason why the theoretical sampling distribution of *r* cannot be applied in Q-contexts is that the statistical model of correlation presumes that any two distributions (of Q-items) taken at random will correlate zero, on the average, with each other. In fact, however, any two randomly-selected Q-sorts may well have a non-zero relationship, on the average, with each other. The statistical model requires a null point, namely a correlation coefficient of zero, around which sampling fluctuations occur. When a correlation is found that is not reasonably acceptable as a sampling fluctuation, then it is deemed "significant." With

person-correlations, however, the null point may *not* be a correlation coefficient of zero and, indeed, is usually unknown. Certain
universally applicable items may be contained in the Q-set
which build in a positive correlation among people. Or the
groups being studied may have certain homogeneities which
tend to create positive inter-person correlations.

In practice the null point has never been generally established
for any Q-set, including the CQ-set. Such an undertaking would
require first a very arbitrary delineation of the universe of
potential subjects of the Q-set followed by massive and enduring
labors of data collection and analysis. Because of the arbitrariness
of the initial definition of a subject domain, this effort at its end
might well not be acceptable as definitive. Since the questions
of inference that such an empirically established sampling distribution of inter-person correlations would intend to serve can be
dealt with alternatively, the whole issue can be avoided by
resort at the outset to these alternative procedures. If we recognize r to be simply a convenient index or score and use statistical
methods appropriate to the obtained distribution of these scores,
we shall be in no danger of making unwarranted inferences. For
the central application we describe now, no problems are created
by this decision.

A primary use of the index of similarity is with regard to the
question, do members of one group correlate higher than members of another group with a criterion? For example, a hypothesis
may be that women coming to an orthopedist with complaints
of low back pain are more hysteric than women coming with
another kind of orthopedic difficulty. In order to test this
hypothesis, it is required first that reliable, consensually based
Q-sorts be established for each of the women in each of the
groups. Second, the concept of "hysteria" must be defined, also
in Q-sort terms. A number of knowledgeable psychiatrists could,
working independently, each Q-sort "the hysterical personality"
by means of the CQ-set. Unquestionably, they would agree
sufficiently to permit the consensual Q-sort derived from their
separate Q-sorts to have a high reproducibility. It is fair to say
that the concept of hysteria is nothing more than what a group of
competent psychiatrists say it is, and so the usual criterion prob-

lem is solved here in a sufficient fashion. Now, the Q-sorts describing the women with low back pain and the Q-sorts describing the women with other orthopedic difficulties are each correlated with the Q-sort expressed definition by psychiatrists of hysteria. By the hypothesis, it would be expected that the average "score" (correlation with the Q-definition of hysteria) for the low back pain group would be higher than the average "score" for the control group. In order to evaluate this hypothesis, the *t*-test or the Mann-Whitney test could be employed, depending on the properties of the distribution of "scores." This general design has wide utility and has already offered some interesting results.

As another illustration of this approach, there is the study by Shapiro (1957). He was interested, among other things, in seeing whether psychological tests predict better for certain types of subjects than they do for others. Representatives of four different types of personality were identified. To serve as criteria, Q-sort formulations of each of these subjects were established by a consensus of psychologists each of whom had had an opportunity to observe the subjects directly in a variety of social and interview settings. The Rorschach protocols of these subjects were then given to experienced psychologists, each of whom expressed by means of a Q-sort his interpretation of the subject as seen through the test. From the multiple interpretations of each subject's Rorschach a consensual Q-sort interpretation was derived. By correlating these consensus interpretations with the criterion definitions of each subject, a score was achieved that reflected the extent to which the test could be said to predict the personality of the subject. By the use of a number of representatives of each personality type, a set of experimentally independent scores was developed for each personality category. Shapiro was then able to test whether members of one personality category are more readily predictable by the Rorschach than are members of another personality category, by testing whether the average of the accuracy scores which characterize one kind of personality was significantly higher (or lower) than the average accuracy score for personalities of another type. In this study, the *r*'s have a different meaning than the *r*'s in the previously described study of women with low back pain. But again, by the use of independent replications, a basis for statistical inference is established which permits proper test of the hypothesis under consideration.

A variety of additional applications of Q-correlations treated as scores can be elaborated. Such questions as the relative homogeneity of groups, the significance of agreement between sorters in describing a set of subjects, the significance of a change in correlation from one time or situation to another, are illustrative. We shall avoid discussing these here for each of these applications is a rather special one, involving much and intricate detail in exposition. Inevitably, a general discussion would prove insufficient as a guide for the specialized applications which are possible, and so the advice is offered that a statistical consultant be called in if these latter or related problems are germane to research. The fundamental consideration to be remembered, however, in developing evaluative procedures for r is that when sets of inter-person correlations are to be statistically evaluated as scores, these r's must be independent of each other. This was true in the hypothetical study of low back pain and hysteria—the correlations with the Q-definition of hysteria are independent of each other for the Q-definition is a constant. This was true also in the Shapiro study cited, where the correlations employed as scores were independent operationally. Unless the scores are independent, the conventional statistical methods do not apply.

Changing direction now, we note that investigators have found it useful to single out individuals for study on the basis of one Q-variable or on the basis of a score on a selected subset of Q-items. For example, "over-controlled" and "under-controlled" individuals may be selected on the basis of just one Q-item or on the basis of a score compiled by summing the values of a number of items designated or previously found to be related to over- and under-control.

A generally better way of placing individuals along a dimension is to first describe, in full Q-sort terms, the hypothetical individuals at each end of the continuum of concern. Then, by correlating the actual Q-sorts of subjects with these conceptual definitions of the dimensional extremes, "scores" are derived which nicely arrange the subjects along the continuum. This method is better than the single variable basis for dimensionalizing individuals because the definition of the dimension is a far richer one and the placement of subjects is based upon 100 Q-items rather than a single one. The method is superior to the procedure of scoring a special cluster of Q-items primarily in regard to convenience and flexibility. Correlations are rapid, cheap, and can proceed automatically. Scoring a subgroup of items cannot be so easily automated for it involves selective search through the complete Q-set and often transformations of item direction so that summing is appropriate. Empirically, in some limited tests, the scores derived from scoring subgroups of Q-items have proven to be functionally interchangeable with scores derived by correlating Q-sorts with Q-definitions of the dimension.

THE INTERCORRELATIONS OF Q-SORTS TO PERMIT, VIA FACTOR OR CLUSTER ANALYSIS, THE DISCERNMENT OF TYPES OR CLUSTERS OF PEOPLE

For many purposes, it may be desirable to go beyond the simple correlation of Q-sorts to the analysis of *matrices* of Q-sort correlations. We may be interested in developing an empirical typology of schizophrenia (Beck, 1954; Guertin & Jenkins, 1956), or of psychiatric inpatients in general (Monro, 1955), or of Air Force officers (Block, 1954), or of the images of psychotherapists held by prospective patients (Apfelbaum, 1958), or of role behaviors (Block, 1952a). Rather than grouping people on some independent basis of classification and then analyzing the characteristics of the Q-sorts that come out of each group, we may reverse the sequence and group individuals on the basis of their Q-sorts, then analyzing independent sources of information for the correlates of group membership. For exploratory studies especially, when we do not already possess a schema with which to view the world, this latter approach is valuable. The techniques primarily used for grouping individuals are factor and cluster analysis.

Factor and cluster analysis—the analysis of communal variance —are by now widely applied and largely understood methods. They are most useful when large masses of data, data too extensive and intertwined to permit of immediate understanding, must be dealt with by an investigator, and it is desired to simplify or group or reduce the number of variables or concepts that must be held in mind. The different methods of analysis may be reviewed in a number of texts and articles, e.g., Guilford, 1954; Fruchter, 1954; Tryon, 1958. Most recently, Tryon (1959) has written an important paper which integrates into one coherent framework the several alternative methods for the analysis of communality. Presently, it can be said that so far as the various dimension-finding procedures are concerned, psychologically equivalent results almost invariably will obtain regardless of the specific method employed. More important than a choice among these methods is a validation or support of the groupings any of these methods provides. Communality analysis is an aid to, not a substitute for incisive conceptualization; it can mislead as it simplifies. Thoughtfully applied and interpreted, however, factor and cluster analytic methods are powerful devices for structuring cogently sets or relationships otherwise impossible to encompass.

Electronic computers have been an additional reason for the development of this field. The advent of high-speed computing machinery has meant that these techniques for perceiving an order in a seeming chaos are suddenly most available. The extended computational labors the analysis of communality has will identify this general influence and permit the investigator, at entailed in the past are now performed by the machines rapidly, accurately, and inexpensively. A large number of research questions that previously were impractical in factor or cluster analytic terms can now be approached by these means.

With specific reference to the factor or cluster analysis of Q-sort data, there are no special complications. The methods can be applied directly and without complication to correlations based upon these data. Although we are using correlation coefficients, the r's we cautioned about in the last section, as the basis for analysis, these correlations are being used in a descriptive sense rather than in connection with questions of statistical inference.

Should there exist a certain intercorrelation among all Q-sorts as a reflection of a "universals" factor, the factor or cluster methods his option, to include or to partial out this contribution to covariation.

A much larger question, to which we have already alluded in Chapter 2, has to do with the general logic of the factor analysis of Q-data rather than its mechanics. Over the years there has been a difference of opinion on the usefulness of correlating people as compared with the correlation cf variables or items. This controversy began between Stephenson (1935) and Burt (1937), was extended by them into a full-scale debate (Burt & Stephenson, 1939) and was joined in by others (Cattell, 1952; Cronbach, 1953; Eysenck, 1954; Block, 1955b). The issue has been whether correlating persons across variables (Q-items) provides any kind of result not completely achievable by means of the traditional approach of correlating variables across people. The correlation of persons orientation, which springs from a "person-centered" emphasis (cf. Ch. 2), was named by Burt as the Q approach; the preference for the correlation of variables, which can be identified with the "variable-centered" attitude, he designated as the R approach.

At this point, it is clear that the issue, which has perseverated over the years, is an empirical one and not, as had been presupposed, solely of a mathematical nature. The available empirical evidence on the question is not yet voluminous but where the comparative approach has been tried (e.g., Block, 1955b; Lorr, Jenkins & Medland, 1955; Block, 1957c) it seems clear that different results are achieved by Q and by R. Indeed, many of the apparent contradictions in the research literature perhaps are understandable as due to the application of an R perspective when the Q approach would have provided coherent results. The reason why so strong an assertion can be made is that the correlation between variables is a function of the sample of individuals on which the data are based. Samples of subjects from one study to another may be differently composed so that a type of personality frequently represented in one research may be absent or atypical in the samples employed by another study. Consequently, the correlations betwen variables can appear to fluctuate wildly from study to study where a respect for the different patterns of personality organization within each of the aggregated samples would reveal the consistent findings toward which we aspire. The reader interested in a larger perspective on this controversy will wish to refer to Cronbach's discussion of "the place of correlation between persons in science" (1953).

Let us presume then that a factor analysis or cluster analysis of Q-correlations has been performed, with the result that a sample of individuals is partitioned into several sub-groups. We may be analyzing the Q-sorts describing the mothers of schizophrenic children (Block, J. H., Patterson, Virginia, Block, J., & Jackson, 1958) or we may be interested in alternative conceptions of adjustment held by different schools of psychotherapy or we may wish to ascertain the kinds of personality and their frequency of representation in a particular business or profession. Given the several subgroups established by factor or cluster analysis, the investigator may wish to put three questions to his data.

He may wish to know just what each of the subgroups is like, in Q-sort terms. The individuals have been grouped on the basis of their Q-sort similarities but after the grouping has been established by the mathematics of the technique, it is of interest to examine the content of the Q-sorts, to form an idea of just what the individuals in a given subgroup are like. If there was a Q-sort of the typical individual in the subgroup, we could simply inspect the items describing this modal character and by their nature directly understand the personality homogeneities that define the subgroup.

What is needed then is a method for establishing a Q-sort known as a "factor-array" that "best represents" all the individuals in the subgroup, for usually no one Q-sort in the subgroup is a sufficiently "pure" representative of the underlying personality category. The simplest and a quite adequate method of constructing a Q-sort which best exemplifies the personality type is to sum, for each item, the Q-values over all the individuals included in the subgroup. For the CQ-set, 100 such sums would be derived and in interpretation, the highest and lowest sums would indicate the Q-items most crucial in defining the modal personality of the subgroup. Obviously, this method of developing a factor-array has the same rationale as the method of pooling judges' evaluations previously described (Chapter 2).[31] Once the factor-array is derived, perusal of the salient (and non-salient) Q-items defining the array readily reveals the psychological meaning of the factor.

Sometimes, it is desirable to compare the Q-sort array representative of one factor or cluster type with the Q-sort array typifying another factor-based group, in order to identify the distinguishing items. Since the factor-arrays to be compared may not be based upon the same number of individuals, comparisons of item sums is confusing and so item *means* should be calculated.

Contrast of two factor-arrays is especially informative for the differences between factors then are to be seen most sharply. In comparing two factor-arrays, no statistical test is appropriate[32] nor is one, in fact, needed. The largest differences in the means of corresponding items may be viewed as discriminating the two factors.

In achieving understanding of the CQ-items distinguished by this "contrast method," it is useful to keep in mind also the *absolute* placement of these items. An item that is "relatively characteristic" of one group may, in the absolute scaling terms in which the Q-sorts were initially expressed, clearly be *uncharacteristic* of the individuals in the group. For example, the CQ-item, "Has warmth; has the capacity for close relationships, compassionate" may discriminate between factor-arrays A and B but in *both* arrays, the mean placement for that item may be *below* the mid-point of the nine-interval judgment continuum. For both Factor A and Factor B, then, "warmth" is a negatively salient or uncharacteristic quality but one group, A, is less extremely viewed than the other, B. Although strictly, this CQ-item is indeed *relatively* characteristic of A in this comparison, it makes

---

[31] When the number of Q-sorts defining a factor is small, it may be worthwhile to employ Spearman's differential weighting procedure. A table to simplify finding the required weights in constructing a factor-array is available in an article by Creaser (1955).

[32] For the different placement of items is the *prior* basis for establishing different factor-types.

better sense in the interpretation to take account also of the absolute position of the item.

When factor-arrays are to be correlated with each other or with other Q-sorts, or when a number of factor-arrays are to be contrasted, it is convenient for the many calculations to be performed clerically, to "re-Q" the distribution of item sums. For the CQ-set, the items with the five highest sums are given scores of 9, the items with the eight next highest sums are awarded scores of 8, the items with the twelve next highest sums are given scores of 7, and so on through the CQ-distribution. By converting item sums to a nine-point score distribution, the factor-arrays effectively are made into Q-sorts. Correlations of these "re-Q'ed" factor-arrays with other Q-sorts may then be calculated by the short-cut method described earlier. Contrasting "re-Q'ed" factor-arrays can proceed most rapidly, by noting the items which, in the commensurate arrays now being compared, are placed in categories discrepant by two or three or four intervals.[33]

A second concern the investigator may wish to investigate is whether persons in one group are different from persons in another group in regard to their scores on other variables or their frequency of placement in other categories. Do individuals of personality type A score differently on a questionnaire or have higher incomes than do individuals of personality type B? Are members of one factor-based group more likely to be Republians or paranoid than are members of another factor-based category? It is of course required that the variables or categories to be related to the factor-based groupings are independent of the Q-data. Otherwise, obtained relationships may reflect only a bootstrap operation. The differences between factor-based groups with regard to non-Q variables are easily evaluated parametrically

---

[33] In "re-Qing" a distribution of item sums, it sometimes happens that several items have the same sum and, by virtue of the fixed number of items to be placed into each category, not all of the tied items can go into a given category. In this situation, perhaps the fairest solution is to assign the tied items to categories on a random basis. It may be worthwhile, however, in inspecting for differences, to remember which items have been assigned in this arbitrary way. For correlational purposes, the random assignment into adjacent categories of the very few Q-items that are involved is unimportant.

by means of the *t-* or *F*-test, depending on whether two or more than two groups are being contrasted. Where non-parametric methods are best used, the Mann-Whitney or Kruskal-Wallis test may be employed. When the relative frequency of factor-based groups in non-Q categories is at issue, the Chi-square test is convenient. All of these methods are described in the references previously cited (p. 109).

A third question the investigator may wish to ask is related to the preceding one but is subtly different and must be answered differently. Sometimes, a Q factor analysis is carried through on two or more *merged* samples of individuals. A sample of mothers of schizophrenic children may be merged with a sample of mothers of neurotic children and then analyzed into types of mothers. A sample of architects may be merged with a sample of engineers and a sample of artists, the total group then being subject to a Q factor or cluster analysis. A question that is of interest to ask after such an analysis is, Are certain of the types found more likely to be made up of individuals from one of the samples than would be expected on the basis of chance? If personality type A consists of 14 architects, 5 engineers and 6 artists, can we say that this type especially includes architects or could such a pattern of membership in this personality category be understood as chance?

The system of probabilities which applies here is known as the *hypergeometric distribution* and may be reviewed in Feller (1957, pp. 41-45) or equivalent sources. Because an explanation of the hypergeometric distribution here would prove burdensome to most readers who may not find occasion to require this information, the formulas involved are not listed here. For the present purposes, it is only important that the precise form of the question answered by the hypergeometric distribution be understood and that a suitable reference for the method be available.

SOME ADDITIONAL SUGGESTIONS

Besides the ways and means already described, some additional usages warrant mention here. These suggestions are more in the way of remarks on possible variations rather than on new categories of application.

For certain kinds of research, it is rather difficult to find a sufficient number of subjects meeting defined criteria. A particular clinic or assessment center simply may not encounter enough individuals with the desired characteristics. If a number of institutions cooperate, however, the required number of subjects often may be accumulated readily. If Q-sort data are of interest, and the Q-sorts are established as reliable and consensually reproducible, then there is no reason why Q-data collected at several places cannot be merged. Samples are thus achieved that otherwise cannot be collected in a reasonable time.

The merging into one sample of individuals Q-sorted by different sets of clinicians is justified because, as ipsative scores, Q-values are not "sample-bound." An individual's Q-values are *not* established by referring him to a particular group of subjects serving as a frame of reference. Rather, the nature of the technique requires that each individual be portrayed in his own right and not *vis-a-vis* a specific reference group.

This opportunity the Q-sort procedure provides, of merging and comparing data from different samples, is a most important facility for the researcher to remember. When this option is properly employed, the generality of results can be investigated extensively. Rival interpretations, equally tenable within one sample, may be tested by adding samples chosen to exclude certain of the competing hypotheses. By such means, findings are achieved that are both more definitive and richer in meaning.

Another kind of application of the Q-sort is in connection with studies where the conceptualizations or interests of the investigators change after the basic data have been collected, e.g., in longitudinal or assessment research. Often, in such studies, subjects are not evaluated at the time of their availability with respect to certain variables or concepts that later appear to be important. It may not be possible to redeem this deficiency directly for subjects may be unavailable for restudy or they may be twenty years older. Retrospective evaluations probably cannot be gathered in any trustworthy way for the memories of judges may be faulty or irremediably affected by other information. Indeed, the originally participating judges may no longer be available.

In such circumstances, if individuals in the subject sample already have been described by means of consensus Q-sorts, their belated "scores" on the omitted variable or concept can be obtained easily by an application of a design previously described. A number of qualified judges would formulate the new concept or the personality implications of the concept in Q-sort terms. Their consensual Q-sort of the concept then could serve as a criterion definition of the new variable. By correlating the actual Q-sorts of the now-departed subjects against the just evolved criterion, scores ordering the subjects on this new dimension become available. A high correlation would mean that a subject is placed highly on this new variable or shows congruence with the new concept; a low correlation would mean the converse.

The resourceful researcher may wish to keep this procedure in mind. The method already has been used in a number of research instances and has been found to provide scores after the fact that are equivalent to corresponding scores directly collected when the subjects were evaluated originally. It is required, however, that a comprehensive set of items be employed for the original Q-sorts of the subjects. Otherwise, it may not be possible to build up a fair definition of a complex concept by means of the elements in the Q-set.

Chapter VIII

CONCLUDING REMARKS

Tʜɪs last chapter has no special organization; it serves simply as a place to set down remarks and suggestions not sensibly included in the monograph as it has been structured so far. Among other things, this chapter compares the Q-sort procedure with competitive techniques, the adjective checklist and conventional rating approaches; it describes a Q-set being developed to characterize a person's developmental history; it presents an adjective Q-set for use by non-professional sorters; and finally, it seeks to give full and proper credit to Stephenson for his methodological innovations and stubborn persistence in quantifying the individual case.

THE Q-SORT AND CHECKLIST PROCEDURES, COMPARED

In a monograph devoted to an application of the Q-sort procedure, the reader perhaps should not expect total objectivity in an evaluation of the relative merits of Q and other methods. Prejudices aside, all of these somewhat overlapping techniques have an unquestionable usefulness. In large part, the superiority we shall (need to) claim for Q-sorting here should be understood as contingent upon a special context of application—judgments by professional observers.

Typically, a checklist consists of a set of adjectives printed on a form. The user simply goes through the list, checking those adjectives he believes to apply to the person he is describing. He may check as many or as few adjectives as he pleases. The task is easy, rapidly-completed and requires no special training. For a given subject, the several checklist descriptions offered by judges are formed into a consensus by noting all the adjectives which have received a predetermined number of checks.

It is not well recognized that checklist approaches and Q-sorting are in some fundamental respects equivalent techniques with equivalent problems. Like the Q-sort method, the checklist procedure is an ipsative technique, i.e., the checklist user describes his subject without reference to a normative comparison group. The adjectives believed to be salient in a positive sense of the person being described are checked. Mention of negatively salient items, however, is not required of the judge and so absence of a check mark is somewhat ambiguous in implication. The unchecked adjective may be irrelevant to the description or it may be informative because it is diametrical to the positively stated picture of the subject.

Like the Q-sort method, the checklist approach imposes a great responsibility upon its developer in collecting and fixing upon a constant set of variables. The adjectives selected must be comprehensive in their descriptive capabilities. The checklist used by judges in research, however, often have been checklists developed primarily for use by lay individuals, e.g., for use in self-descriptions.[34] Consequently, redundancies that are desirable when a checklist is being employed by a lay person may prove to be intolerable when placed in the hands of a sophisticated observer. Large aspects of personality, especially those concerned with matters of which the individual is unaware, cannot be described for the variables needed simply may not be in the collection of adjectives or are not defined well as single adjectives. Presently, no checklist designed for use by professional assessors is available.

The prime differences between the Q-sort and checklist procedures appear to be methodological. Q-sorting collects data in continuous form; the checklist method produces dichotomous data, adjectives checked as applicable and adjectives not checked as applicable. All things else being equal, i.e., with the same number of variables in the item-pool, it is obvious that many more

---

[34] When the contrast between what judges say about a subject and what the subject says about himself is of interest, judges of course must conform to a procedure suitable to the subject.

discriminations are provided by Q-sorting than by the checklist procedure.

The Q-sort technique excludes response sets and order effects where the checklist method is especially susceptible to these disturbing influences. By the use of a *forced* distribution of a *shuffled* set of Q-items, extraneous inter- and intra-judge differences are eliminated. With a checklist, on the other hand, different judges check different numbers of adjectives in characterizing a subject. The *fixed* order in which the list of adjectives is scanned also intrudes an undesirable component for as a judge scans through the printed list of adjectives, significantly large fluctuations in his checking tendency may be observed. These effects are bothersome—freely checking judges are by no means more perceptive but they tend to dominate consensus evaluations; order effects increase the unreliability of the consensus. The rationale for preventing these effects has been discussed earlier, in Chapter VI.

Now, these criticisms—of response sets and order effects in checklist descriptions—can be met. Each adjective can be printed on a separate card and judges may be required to place a specified number of adjectives in each of the two categories. If evaluations more finely graded than dichotomous judgments are desired or are felt to be feasible, then a continuum of discrimination may be imposed upon the judges. And finally, if the adjective set is compiled thoughtfully, we are returned to a full-fledged Q-sort procedure! Regrettably, though, the speed and simplicity of the checklist approach will have been lost.

Questions of speed and simplicity, when professional observers are employed, should be compelling only rarely. If discriminations are achievable, they should be sought; if response sets are undesirable, they should be denied existence. The primary advantage of the checklist approach is its ready acceptance and ease of accomplishment by non-professionals. For this application, checklists have a convenience which often outweighs their methodological deficiencies.

THE Q-SORT AND CONVENTIONAL RATINGS, COMPARED

We have already, in Chapter II and elsewhere, commented in some detail on the relation of Q-sort and conventional rating data. Both methods are devices to permit the expression of judgments, the one being ipsative, the other normative in approach. Both provide data in continuous form. The Q-sort procedure requires a comprehensive set of variables for its effective operation; normative ratings do not have to be exhaustive in coverage. It has been demonstrated that ipsatively-collected Q-data, when treated normatively, contain all the information available through normative ratings (Block, 1957a). If the sample of subjects being evaluated is not so large as to overload the memory of judges, it seems clear that normative ratings can be arranged to perform the same functions available through the Q-sort procedure.

In research settings, the choice of method—ratings or Q-sort—depends on several matters. There is first, perhaps, a conceptual or esthetic preference—for variable-centered versus person-centered data—which may well be all-determining. But practical issues, too, intervene.

If subjects are accumulated slowly, normative ratings prove to depend heavily upon the recall ability of the raters. If ratings are made for each subject separately, the resulting data are ipsative and are susceptible to various response sets. Often, such individual ratings pile up in one or only a few categories, thus providing little discrimination. In such circumstances, there is uncertainty as to whether the apparent homogeneity of the subjects is a genuine finding or is instead an artifact of judge behavior. Compelling judges to employ, with certain frequencies, all the intervals along a rating dimension is a stratagem employed and of course is akin to the forced distribution requirement of Q-sorting.[35]

---

[35] With conventional ratings, this forced spread of judgments has a limitation the importance of which the researcher may wish to evaluate. The opportunity is destroyed of specifying the modal character of a particular research sample where this may provide important contrasts with other research samples. For example, jet pilots happen, as a group, to be evaluated as highly masculine individuals. Forced discrimination among members of this sample with regard to this dimension where

It will often be the case, however, that the decision between conventional ratings and the Q-sort procedure will be based upon questions of research convenience and of research tactics.

The normative rating method clearly has a more immediate convenience since only one variable is dealt with at one time and the subject sample may be readily evaluated in terms of the particular one or two dimensions of interest. To achieve Q-scores on but a few dimensions, *all* of the Q-items must be sorted for *each* subject, a task which may be quite formidable. It should be noted, though, that normative ratings lose this advantage of convenience as the number of variables being rated increases.

Tactically, the Q-sorting of subjects, day-by-day, seems to be less overwhelming for judges than the reckoning they must later face, when the subject sample is complete, of rating rapidly *all* subjects on *all* variables. By the steady accumulation of evaluations via Q, subjects are described and may then be forgotten— a less demanding situation for judges. Moreover, the research is freed from excessive dependence upon the continued availability throughout the study of the judges who observed subjects seen during early phases. When normative ratings are collected over long periods of time, the problem of unavailable judges of unavailable subjects can be a very real one.

DEVELOPING A HISTORICAL Q-SET

In the statement of aims for the CQ-set (Chapter I), it was emphasized that the descriptive procedure was to be applied to characterize a person as he existed and was understood at the time of evaluation. In Lewinian terms, a CQ-description is a contemporaneous one, expressed without regard for the particular circumstances or history of the individual out of which his current personality evolved. The antecedents of personality, however, are no less important than specification of the contemporaneous properties of an individual. By the same logic advanced for the CQ-set, it seems obvious that a carefully

---

little variability exists is a difficult task for the judge and results in unreliable data. It also prevents recognition that members of this sample, on the average, are judged as more masculine than members of a sample, for example, of medical students.

selected, comprehensive set of variables in terms of which a subject's past may be described, would provide a most helpful way of systematizing the historical understanding of an individual.

To this end, work was initiated as early as 1952 to develop a set of Q-variables by means of which an integrated view of a person's developmental history may be expressed. This collection of items has been designated the DQ-procedure.[36]

The Q-sort procedure again seemed an appropriate method to employ for the intent is to order developmentally relevant variables in terms of their salience or decisiveness for the particular individual. Thus, for example, the DQ-item, "Target of some form of ethnocentrism," is perhaps not so salient for a Jew as it is for a Negro in our society. The same item probably is not so decisive for a Catholic living in Boston as it is for a Catholic reared in Oklahoma. We do not consider it sufficient simply to list the determining influence in a person's life. The DQ-procedure aims, in addition, to permit expression of just how the history-viewer unifies and intertwines the multitudinous familial and cultural factors that contribute toward character.

To give a further indication of the content of the DQ-set, we list some additional items: "Mother encouraging and supportive of S's steps toward independence and maturity"; "Father and mother generally shared similar values and orientations"; "Family emphasized 'togetherness', did things as a unit"; "Emphasis in home on manners, propriety and convention"; "Mother was a long-suffering, self-sacrificing, defeated person"; "Paternal emphasis on intellectual achievement"; "Family beset by many tragedies and misfortunes (e.g., illness, death, accidents, radical dislocations. Consider cumulative effect)."

The DQ-set is still in too preliminary a form to warrant circulation currently. It is presently being used and tested in several researches. The resulting data will be studied and the item-set revised before a wider use is encouraged. With the formation of a descriptive complement of the CQ-set, the relations between historical and contemporaneous levels of understanding should

---

[36] The DQ-set is being developed with Jeanne Block.

become open to study in a number of fruitful ways, to test large questions of how individuals happen to evolve toward different character structures.

AN ADJECTIVE Q-SET FOR USE BY
NON-PROFESSIONAL SORTERS

Although the primary purpose of this book has been to present and to justify the Q-sort method for the problem of codifying professional observers, the method continues to have an important application as a research device for use by laymen. For this purpose, it is necessary that the Q-items employed be readily understood by the subject populations it is proposed to study. Various Q-sets for use by non-professionals, for example in self-description procedures, have appeared in the literature (cf., e.g., Butler and Haigh, 1954) and have seen varying degrees of acceptance. For reasons that by now would be repetitious to recite, it clearly would be useful to settle upon one reasonably adequate Q-set for use in such research unless there are strong theoretical reasons to contra-indicate this conformity. However, for various reasons, many of the Q-sort procedures employed in the past with lay subjects may be judged deficient. The Q-items used often have expressed too specialized an orientation or have been highly redundant; use of a large number of items and of categories has tended to make the procedure too demanding of the subject; and undesirable response sets have sometimes been permitted. Reasoning from this analysis, it seems worthwhile, then, to bring forward still another Q-set for research in this domain.

Offered in Appendix H is an adjective Q-set for use by non-professional sorters. It consists of 70 items, to be arranged into seven categories with ten items in each category and is oriented toward comprehensiveness in its coverage of the personality sphere. The item set has evolved in the course of several studies (Block and Thomas, 1955; Chang and Block, 1960; Block and Turula, 1961) and has been further benefited by the suggestions of a number of psychologists.* By virtue of this adjective Q-set's

---

* For their thoughtful considerations here, I am indebted to Bela Baker, Jeanne Block, Elaine Simpson and Donald Woodworth.

history of usefulness in a number of researches, it seems reasonable now to list the adjectives for possible adoption by other researchers.

The uniform distribution suggested for this Q-set, of ten items in each of seven categories, is an easy requirement to communicate to the subject and does not strain his discrimination capacity. In this form, the adjective Q-set may be used as a self-administering procedure with individuals of a high-school educational level. To facilitate this application, there is also included in Appendix H a sample of the instructions employed when the adjective Q-set has been employed as a self-administering procedure in group settings. Subjects typically complete their first sorting of this adjective Q-set in less than thirty minutes. Subsequent sortings require perhaps twenty minutes or so. The procedure does not appear to be an onerous one for the participating subjects.

A CREDIT TO STEPHENSON

There are fads in science as well as in fashion and the letter, Q, has already experienced in psychology its share of unwarranted enthusiasm and unmitigated criticism. Hopefully, as the vanities and hostilities of the moment tire with time or seize upon new objects of passion, and as perspectives accumulate out of experience, the significance of Q for the study of personality may be more objectively evaluated. In any assessment of Q-technique the contribution of William Stephenson cannot be underestimated.

Stephenson, of course, innovated a methodology. His more important service, though, probably has been to insist stubbornly on the possibilities and fruitfulness of quantifying the individual case. By recognizing the different kinds of lawfulness available from variable-centered and from person-centered data, he was able to come forward with a methodology and analytical orientation which has meshed excitingly with the research needs of students of personality.

In our own application of the Q-sort procedure, we have chosen to differ with certain methodological recommendations of Stephenson. In part, these differences stem from a divergence in our respective goals; in part, these differences represent genuine disagreements as to how to proceed. Our intent now, by way of conclusion, is to record the very genuine debt the present effort owes to Stephenson. It is hoped that the present work may bring out for further evaluation and further application the techniques and principles Stephenson has advanced.

REFERENCES

Apfelbaum, B.: *Dimensions of Transference in Psychotherapy*. Berkeley: University of California Press, 1958.

Attneave, F.: *Application of Information theory to Psychology*. New York: Holt-Dryden, 1959.

Barron, F.: Originality in relation to personality and intellect. *J. Pers.*, 1957, *25*:730-742.

Beck, S. J.: The six schizophrenias. *Res. Monogr. Amer. Orthopsychiat. Assn.*, 1954, No. 6.

Block, J.: The assessment of communication: II. Role variations as a function of interactional context. *J. Pers.*, 1952, *21*:272-286. (a)

Block, J.: The Q-sort in assessment and some problems in its use. *IPAR Research Bulletin*, 1952. (b)

Block, J.: A differentiated approach to the officer selection problem. *IPAR Research Report*. Prepared under Contract No. AF 18 (600)-8. 1954.

Block, J.: Personality characteristics associated with fathers' attitudes toward child-rearing. *Child Develpm.*, 1955, *26*:41-48. (a)

Block, J.: The difference between Q and R. *Psychol. Rev.*, 1955, *62*: 356-358. (b)

Block, J.: A comparison of the forced and unforced Q-sorting procedures. *Educ. Psychol. Measmt.*, 1956, *16*:481-493.

Block, J.: A comparison between ipsative and normative ratings of personality. *J. Abnorm. & Social Psychol.*, 1957, *54*:50-54. (a)

Block, J.: Studies in the phenomenology of emotions. *J. Abnorm. & Social Psychol.*, 1957, *54*:358-363. (b)

Block, J.: A study of affective responsiveness in a lie-detection situation. *J. Abnorm. & Social Psychol.*, 1957, *55*:11-15. (c)

Block, J.: On the number of significant findings to be expected from chance. *Psychometrika*, 1960, *25*: 369-380.

Block, J., and Bailey, D. E.: Q-sort item analyses of a number of MMPI measures of personality, interest and intellect. *IPAR Research Report*. Prepared under Contract No. AF 18 (600)—8, 1954.

Block, J., and Bailey, D. E.: Q-sort item analyses of a number of MMPI scales. *Technical Memorandum* OERL TM-55-7. Maxwell Air Force Base, Alabama: Officer Education Research Laboratory, May 1955.

Block, J., and Bennett, Lillian: The assessment of communication: perception and transmission as a function of the social situation. *Human Relat.*, 1955, 8:317-325.

Block, J., and Gough, H. G.: An application of the Q-sort technique to the California Psychological Inventory. *Technical Memorandum* OERL TM-55-8. Maxwell Air Force Base, Alabama: Officer Edu· cation Research Laboratory, May 1955.

Block, J., and Petersen, P.: Some personality correlates of confidence, caution and speed in a decision situation. *J. Abnorm. & Social Psychol.*, 1955, *51*: 34-41. (a)

Block, J., and Petersen, P.: Q-sort item analyses of a number of Strong Vocational Interest Inventory scales. *Technical Memorandum* OERL TM-55-9, Maxwell Air Force Base, Alabama: Officer Education Research Laboratory, May 1955. (b)

Block, J. and Thomas, H.: Is satisfaction with self a measure of adjustment? *J. abnorm. soc. Psychol.*, *51*, 254-259, 1955.

Block, J. and Turula, Emily: Identification, ego-control and adjustment. Unpublished manuscript, 1961.

Block, Jeanne, Patterson, V. L., Block, J., and Jackson, D. D.: A study of the parents of schizophrenic and neurotic children. *Psychiatry*, 1958, *21*:387-397.

Borland, L., and Hardyck, C.: Personality characteristics associated with the use of hypnosis in dental practice. Unpublished manuscript, 1960.

Burt, C.: Correlations between persons. *Brit. J. Psychol.*, 1937, *28*:59-96.

Burt, C., and Stephenson, W.: Alternative views on correlation between persons. *Psychometrika*, 1939, *4*:269-281.

Butler, J. M. and Haigh, G. V.: Changes in the relation between self-concepts and ideal concepts consequent upon client-centered counseling. In C. R. Rogers and Rosalind F. Dymond (Eds.), *Psychotherapy and personality change*. Univ. of Chicago Press, 1954, pp. 55-76.

Campbell, D. T., and Fiske, D. M.: Convergent and discriminant validation by the multitrait-multimethod matrix. *Psychol. Bull.*, 1959, *56*:81-105.

Cattell, R. B.: Psychological measurement: ipsative, normative, and interactive. *Psychol. Rev.*, 1944, *51*:292-303.

Cattell, R. B.: The three basic factor-analytic research designs—their interrelations and derivatives. *Psychol. Bull.*, 1952, *49*:499-520.

Chang, Judy and Block, J.: A study of identification in male homosexuals. *J. consult. Psychol.*, *24*, 307-310, 1960.

Clark, E. L.: Spearman-Brown formula applied to ratings of personality traits. *J. educ. Psychol.*, 1935, *26*:552-555.

Cohen, J.: An aid in the computation of correlation based on Q sorts. *Psychol. Bull.*, 1957, *54*:138-139.

Creaser, J.: An aid in calculating Q-sort factor arrays. *J. clin. Psychol.*, 1955, *11*: 195-196.

Cronbach, L. J.: Further evidence on response-sets and test design. *Educ. psychol. Measmt*, 1950, *10*: 3-31.

Cronbach, L. J.: Correlations between persons as a research tool. In O. H. Mowrer (Ed.), *Psychotherapy Theory and Research*. New York: Ronald Press, 1953, pp. 376-388. (a)

Cronbach, L. J.: *A consideration of information theory and utility theory as tools for psychometic problems*. Urbana, Ill.: Coll. of Educ., University of Illiois, 1953. (b)

Cronbach, L. J., and Gleser, Goldine C.: Assessing similarity between profiles. *Psychol. Bull.*, 1953, *50*:456-473.

Cronbach, L. J., and Gleser, Goldine. Book review of Stephenson, W. *The study of behavior*. *Psychometrika*, 1954, *19*:327-331.

Cronbach, L. J., and Meehl, P. E. Construct validity in psychological tests. *Psychol. Bull.*, 1955, *52*:281-302.

Crutchfield, R. S.: Conformity and character. *Amer. Psychologist*, 1955, *10*:191-198.

Crutchfield, R. S., Woodworth, D. G. and Albrecht, Ruth E.: Perceptual performance and the effective person. Lackland Air Force Base, Tex.: Personnel Laboratory, Wright Air Development Center, April 1958. (*Technical Report* WADC—TN—58—60 ASTIA Document No. AD 151 039.)

Dalaba, O. G.: A development study of ego-control. Doctoral dissertation, Univer. of California, Berkeley, 1960.

Dingman, H F., and Guilford, J. P.: A new method for obtaining weighted composites of ratings. *J. appl. Psychol.*, 1954, *38*:305-307.

Dunnette, M. D., and Hoggatt, A. C.: Deriving a composite score from several measures of the same attribute. *Educ. psychol. Measmt*, 1957, *17*:423-434.

Edwards, A.: Social desirability and Q sorts. *J. consult. Psychol.*, 1955, *19*:462.

Enright, J. B.: Profile types and prediction from the *Minnesota Multiphasic Personality Inventory.* Doctoral dissertation, Univer. of California, Berkeley, 1959.

Eriksen, C. W., and Davids, A.: The meaning and clinical validity of the Taylor Anxiety Scale and the Hysteria-Psychasthemia Scales from the MMPI. *J. Abnorm. & Social Psychol.*, 1955, *50*:135-137.

Eriksen, C. W., and Browne, C. T.: An experimental and theoretical analysis of perceptual defense. *J. Abnorm. & Social Psychol.*, 1956, *52*:224-230.

Eysenck, H. J.: The science of personality: nomothetic! *Psychol. Rev.*, 1954, *61*:339-342.

Feller, W.: *An Introduction to Probability Theory and Its Applications.* (2nd ed.) Vol. 1. New York: Wiley, 1957.

Ferguson, G. A.: On the theory of test discrimination. *Psychometrika*, 1949, *14*:61-68.

Forer, B. R., and Tolman, Ruth S.: Some characteristics of clinical judgment. *J. consult. Psychol.*, 1952, *16*:347-352.

Frank, G. H.: Note on the reliability of Q-sort data. *Psychol. Rep.*, 1956, *2*:182.

Fruchter, B.: *Introduction to Factor Analysis.* New York: Van Nostrand, 1954.

Goodling, R. A., and Guthrie, G. M.: Some practical considerations in Q-sort item selection. *J. counsel. Psychol.*, 1956, *3*:70-72.

Gordon, Kate: Group judgments in the field of lifted weights. *J. exp. Psychol.*, 1924, *7*:398-400.

Gough, H. G.: The adjective check list as a personality assessment research technique. *Psychol. Reports*, 1960, *6*:107-122.

Guertin, W. H., and Jenkins, R. L.: A transposed factor analysis of a group of schizophrenic patients. *J. clin. Psychol.*, 1956, *12*:64-68.

Guilford, J. P.: *Psychometric Methods.* New York: McGraw-Hill, 1954.

Haggard, E. A.: *Intraclass Correlation and the Analysis of Variance.* New York: Dryden, 1958.

Halbower, C. C.: A comparison of actuarial vs. clinical predictions to classes discriminated by the MMPI. Doctoral dissertation. Univer. of Minnesota, 1955.

Hilden, A. H.: *Manual for Q-sort and Random Sets of Personal Concepts.* Webster Groves 19, Mo. (628 Clark Ave.): Author 1954.

Hilden, A. H.: Q-sort correlation: stability and random choice of statements. *J. consult Psychol.,* 1958, *22:*45-50.

Holt, R. R.: Clinical and statistical prediction: a reformulation and some new data. *J. Abnorm. & Social Psychol.,* 1958, *56:*1-12.

Horst, P.: Obtaining a composite measure from a number of different measures of the same attribute. *Psychometrika,* 1936, *1:*53-60.

Hotelling, H.: Analysis of a complex of statistical variables into principal components. *J. educ. Psychol.,* 1933, *24:*417-441.

Jackson, D. D., Block, Jack, Block, Jeanne, and Patterson, V.: Psychiatrists' conception of the schizophrenogenic parent. *Arch. Neurol. Psychiat.,* 1958, *79:*448-459.

Jones, M. B.: Composite ratings and the case of unit rank. *J. appl. Psychol.,* 1957, *41:*198-200.

Kelley, E. L., and Fiske, D. W.: *The Prediction of Performance in Clinical Psychology.* Ann Arbor: Univer. of Michigan Press, 1951.

Kemeny, J. G.: Mathematics without numbers. *Daedalus,* 1959, *88:* 577-591.

Kerr, W. A., and Speroff, B. J.: *The Empathy Test.* Chicago: Psychometric Affiliates, 1951.

Knupfer, Genevieve, Jackson, D. D., and Krieger, G.: Personality differences between more and less competent psychotherapists as a function of criteria of competence. *J. Nerv. Ment. Dis.,* 1959, *129:* 375-384.

Kruskal, W. H., and Wallis, W. A.: Use of ranks in one-criterion variance analysis. *J. Amer. Statist. Assn.,* 1952, *47:*583-621.

Lawshe, C. H., and Nagle, B. F.: A note on the combination of ratings on the basis of reliability. *Psychol. Bull.,* 1952, *49:*270-273.

Lewin, K.: Defining the "field at a given time." *Psychol. Rev.,* 1943, *50:*292-310.

Livson, N. H., and Nichols, T. F.: Discrimination and reliability in Q-sort personality descriptions. *J. Abnorm. & Social Psychol.,* 1956, *52:*159-165.

Lorr, M.: Multidimensional scale for rating psychiatric patients. Hospital form. *Vet. Adm. Tech. Bull.,* 10-507, Nov. 1953.

Lorr, M., Jenkins, R., and Medland, F. F.: Direct versus obserse factor analysis: a comparison of results. *Educ. Psychol. Measmt.,* 1955, *15:*441-449.

MacKinnon, D. W., *et al:* An assessment study of Air Force officers: Part I. Design of the study and description of the variables. Lackland Air Force Base, Tex.: Personnel Laboratory, Wright Air Development Center, 1958. (*Technical Report* WADC-TN-58-91, Part I, ASTIA Document No. AD 152 040.)

Mann, H. B., and Whitney, D. R.: On a test of whether one of two random variables is stochastically larger than the other. *Ann. Math. Statist.*, 1947, *18*:50-60.

McCornack, R. L.: A criticism of studies comparing item weighting methods. *J. appl. Psychol.*, 1956, *40*:343-344.

McHugh, R. B.: The criterial estimation of a true score. *Psychol. Bull.*, 1957, *54*:73-74.

McNemar, Q.: *Psychological Statistics.* (2nd ed.) New York: Wiley, 1955.

McReynolds, P., Ballachey, E., and Ferguson, J. T.: Development and evaluation of a behavioral scale for appraising the adjustment of hospitalized patients. *Amer. Psychologist,* 1952, *7*:340.

Meehl, P. E.: Wanted—a good cookbook. *Amer. Psychologist,* 1956, *11*:263-272.

Monro, A. B.: Psychiatric types: a Q-technique study of 200 patients. *J. ment. Sci.,* 1955, *101*:330-343.

Mowrer, O. H.: "Q-technique"—description, history and critique. In O. H. Mowrer (Ed.), *Psychotherapy Theory and Research.* New York: Ronald Press, 1953, pp. 316-375.

Murray, H. A.: *Explorations in Personality.* New York: Oxford Univ. Press, 1938.

Polansky, N. A.: How shall a life history be written? *Charact. & Pers.,* 1941, *9*:188-207.

Rajaratnam, N., Cronbach, L. J., and Gleser, Goldine C.: Reliability as generalizability. Mimeographed. Bureau of Educational Research, Univer. of Illinois, 1960.

Reichenbach, H.: *The Rise of Scientific Philosophy.* Berkeley: Univer. of California Press, 1951.

Remmers, H. H.: The equivalence of judgments to test items in the sense of the Spearman-Brown formula. *J. Educ. Psychol.,* 1931, *22*:66-71.

Rosander, A. C.: The Spearman-Brown formula in attitude scale construction. *J. Exp. Psychol.,* 1936, *19*:486-495.

Sarbin, T. R., Taft, R., and Bailey, D. E.: *Clinical Inference and Cognitive Theory.* New York: Rinehart, 1960.

Shapiro, A.: Consensus and accuracy of personality appraisals based on test protocols. Doctoral dissertation. Univer. of California, Berkeley, 1957.

Spearman, C.: *The Abilities of Man.* New York: Macmillan, 1927.

Stephenson, W.: Correlating Persons Instead of Tests. *Charact. & Pers.*, 1935, *4*:17-24.

Stephenson, W.: Introduction to inverted factor analysis, with some applications to studies in orexis. *J. educ. Psychol.*, 1936, *27*:353-367.

Stephenson, W.: *The Study of Behavior.* Chicago: Univer. of Chicago Press, 1953.

Thurstone, L. L.: Multiple Factor Analysis. Chicago: Univer. of Chicago Press, 1947.

Tryon, R. C.: Cumulative communality cluster analysis. *Educ. psychol. Measmt.*, 1958, *18*:3-35.

Tryon, R. C.: Domain sampling formulation of cluster and factor analysis. *Psychometrika*, 1959, *24*:113-135.

Twain, D. C.: Factor analysis of a particular aspect of behavioral control: impulsivity. *J. clin. Psychol.*, 1957, *13*:133-136.

Valentine, C. W.: The relative reliability of men and women in intuitive judgments of character. *Brit. J. Psychol.*, 1929, *19*:213-238.

Walker, Helen M., and Lev, J.: *Statistical Inference.* New York: Holt, 1953.

Wilks, S. S.: Weighting systems for linear functions of correlated variables when there is no dependent variable. *Psychometrika*, 1938, *3*:23-40.

Wittenborn, J. R.: Symptom patterns in a group of mental hospital patients. *J. consult. Psychol.*, 1951, *15*:290-302.

Appendix A

THE CALIFORNIA Q-SET (FORM III)

Specified 9-point distribution (N = 100):
5, 8, 12, 16, 18, 16, 12, 8, 5

$$r = 1 - \frac{\text{Sum } d_{ip}^2}{864}$$

1. Is critical, skeptical, not easily impressed.
2. Is a genuinely dependable and responsible person.
3. Has a wide range of interests (N.B. Superficiality or depth of interest is irrelevant here.)
4. Is a talkative individual.
5. Behaves in a giving way toward others. (N.B. regardless of the motivation involved.)
6. Is fastidious.
7. Favors conservative values in a variety of areas.
8. Appears to have a high degree of intellectual capacity. (N.B. whether actualized or not.) (N.B. Originality is not necessarily assumed.)
9. Is uncomfortable with uncertainty and complexities.
10. Anxiety and tension find outlet in bodily symptoms. (N.B. If placed high, implies bodily dysfunction; if placed low, implies absence of autonomic arousal.)
11. Is protective of those close to him. (N.B. Placement of this item expresses behavior ranging from over-protection through appropriate nurturance to a laissez-faire, under-protective manner.)
12. Tends to be self-defensive.
13. Is thin-skinned; sensitive to anything that can be construed as criticism or an interpersonal slight.
14. *Genuinely* submissive; accepts domination comfortably.
15. Is skilled in social techniques of imaginative play, pretending and humor.

16. Is introspective and concerned with self as an object. (N.B. introspectiveness *per se* does not imply insight.)
17. Behaves in a sympathetic or considerate manner.
18. Initiates humor.
19. Seeks reassurance from others.
20. Has a rapid personal tempo; behaves and acts quickly.
21. Arouses nurturant feelings in others.
22. Feels a lack of personal meaning in life.
23. Extrapunitive; tends to transfer or project blame.
24. Prides self on being "objective," rational.
25. Tends toward over-control of needs and impulses; binds tensions excessively; delays gratification unnecessarily.
26. Is productive; gets things done.
27. Shows condescending behavior in relations with others. (N.B. Extreme placement toward uncharacteristic end implies simply an *absence* of condescension, not necessarily equalitarianism or inferiority.)
28. Tends to arouse liking and acceptance in people.
29. Is turned to for advice and reassurance.
30. Gives up and withdraws where possible in the face of frustration and adversity. (N.B. If placed high, implies generally defeatist; if placed low, implies *counteractive.*)
31. Regards self as physically attractive.
32. Seems to be aware of the impression he makes on others.
33. Is calm, relaxed in manner.
34. Over-reactive to minor frustrations; irritable.
35. Has warmth; has the capacity for close relationships; compassionate
36. Is subtly negativistic; tends to undermine and obstruct or sabotage.
37. Is guileful and deceitful, manipulative, opportunistic.
38. Has hostility towards others. (N.B. Basic hostility is intended here; mode of expression is to be indicated by other items.)
39. Thinks and associates to ideas in unusual ways; has unconventional thought processes.
40. Is vulnerable to real or fancied threat, generally fearful.
41. Is moralistic. (N.B. Regardless of the particular nature of the moral code.)

42. Reluctant to commit self to any definite course of action; tends to delay or avoid action.
43. Is facially and/or gesturally expressive.
44. Evaluates the motivation of others in interpreting situations. (N.B. Accuracy of evaluation is not assumed.) (N.B. again. Extreme placement in one direction implies pre-occupation with motivational interpretation; at the other extreme, the item implies a psychological obtuseness, S does not consider motivational factors.)
45. Has a brittle ego-defense system; has a small reserve of integration; would be disorganized and maladaptive when under stress or trauma.
46. Engages in personal fantasy and daydreams, fictional speculations.
47. Has a readiness to feel guilty. (N.B. regardless of whether verbalized or not.)
48. Keeps people at a distance; avoids close interpersonal relationships.
49. Is basically distrustful of people in general; questions their motivations.
50. Is unpredictable and changeable in behavior and attitudes.
51. Genuinely values intellectual and cognitive matters. (N.B. Ability or achievement are not implied here.)
52. *Behaves* in an assertive fashion. (N.B. Item 14 reflects underlying submissiveness; this refers to overt behavior.)
53. Various needs tend toward relatively direct and uncontrolled expression; unable to delay gratification.
54. Emphasizes being with others; gregarious.
55. Is self-defeating.
56. Responds to humor.
57. Is an interesting, arresting person.
58. Enjoys sensuous experiences (including touch, taste, smell, physical contact).
59. Is concerned with own body and the adequacy of its physiological functioning.
60. Has insight into own motives and behavior.
61. Creates and exploits dependency in people. (N.B. Regardless of the technique employed, e.g., punitiveness, over-indulgence.) (N.B. At other end of scale, item implies respecting and encouraging the independence and individuality of others.)

62. Tends to be rebellious and non-conforming.
63. Judges self and others in conventional terms like "popularity," "the correct thing to do," social pressures, etc.
64. Is socially perceptive of a wide range of interpersonal cues.
65. Characteristically pushes and tries to stretch limits; sees what he can get away with.
66. Enjoys esthetic impressions; is esthetically reactive.
67. Is self-indulgent.
68. Is basically anxious.
69. Is sensitive to anything that can be construed as a demand. (N.B. No implication of the kind of subsequent response is intended here.)
70. *Behaves* in an ethically consistent manner; is consistent with own personal standards.
71. Has high aspiration level for self.
72. Concerned with own adequacy as a person, either at conscious or unconscious levels. (N.B. A clinical judgment is required here; number 74 reflects subjective satisfaction with self.)
73. Tends to perceive many different contexts in sexual terms; eroticizes situations.
74. Is subjectively unaware of self-concern; feels satisfied with self.
75. Has a clear-cut, internally consistent personality. (N.B. *Amount* of information available before sorting is not intended here.)
76. Tends to project his own feelings and motivations onto others.
77. Appears straightforward, forthright, candid in dealing with others.
78. Feels cheated and victimized by life; self-pitying.
79. Tends to ruminate and have persistent, pre-occupying thoughts.
80. Interested in members of the opposite sex. (N.B. At opposite end, item implies *absence* of such interest.)
81. Is physically attractive; good-looking. (N.B. The cultural criterion is to be applied here.)
82. Has fluctuating moods.
83. Able to see to the heart of important problems.
84. Is cheerful. (N.B. Extreme placement toward uncharacteristic end of continuum implies unhappiness or depression.)
85. Emphasizes communication through action and non-verbal behavior.

86. Handles anxiety and conflicts by, in effect, refusing to recognize their presence; repressive or dissociative tendencies.

87. Interprets basically simple and clear-cut situations in complicated and particularizing ways.

88. Is personally charming.

89. Compares self to others. Is alert to real or fancied differences between self and other people.

90. Is concerned with philosophical problems; e.g., religions, values, the meaning of life, etc.

91. Is power oriented; values power in self or others.

92. Has social poise and presence; appears socially at ease.

93a. *Behaves* in a masculine style and manner.

93b. Behaves in a feminine style and manner. (N.B. If subject is male, 93a. applies; if subject is female, 93b. is to be evaluated. (N.B. again. The cultural or sub-cultural conception is to be applied as a criterion.)

94. Expresses hostile feelings directly.

95. Tends to proffer advice.

96. Values own independence and autonomy.

97. Is emotionally bland; has flattened affect.

98. Is verbally fluent; can express ideas well.

99. Is self-dramatizing; histrionic.

100. Does not vary roles; relates to everyone in the same way.

California Q-set Record Sheet

Subject: _____   Sorter: _____   Informational source: _____   Date: _____

1	2	3	4	5	6	7	8	9	10	11	12	13	14	15	16	17	18	19	20

21	22	23	24	25	26	27	28	29	30	31	32	33	34	35	36	37	38	39	40

41	42	43	44	45	46	47	48	49	50	51	52	53	54	55	56	57	58	59	60

61	62	63	64	65	66	67	68	69	70	71	72	73	74	75	76	77	78	79	80

81	82	83	84	85	86	87	88	89	90	91	92	93	94	95	96	97	98	99	100

Specified CQ distribution

Category value	1	2	3	4	5	6	7	8	9
Number of items in category	5	8	12	16	18	16	12	8	5

Formula for correlation between CQ sorts: $r = 1 - \dfrac{\text{sum } d^2}{864}$

N.B. A value of 9 indicates "most characteristic"; a value of 1 indicates "least characteristic".

Appendix B

INSTRUCTIONS FOR USING THE CALIFORNIA Q-SET

Before describing in detail the procedure to be followed in sorting the California Q-set, a few words on the rationale and general purpose of the method are in order.

The non-comparability of clinical formulations because of differences in language usage is a great obstacle to clinical communication and research. Many controversies arise and persist because of this language problem. Thus, clinical interpretations of a patient may differ for two reasons: (1) divergent points of view and analysis, and (2) the basically irrelevant differences in the phrase-making of clinicians. We are interested in the first of these factors, not the second, which operates to confuse the critical issues.

The purpose of the 100 items in the California Q-set is to provide a "Basic English" for clinicians to use in their formulations of individual personalities. Ideally—and the set is not yet ideal—the items should permit the portrayal of any kind of pathology and any kind of normalcy. It is felt that the use of a standard language and procedure permits the descriptions of an individual in a way that is not too atomizing or constraining and by so doing enables comparisons to be made which otherwise could not be achieved.

The procedure is essentially simple, if somewhat cumbersome. With the individual to be "formulated" in mind, look through the 100 cards. You are to sort these statements into a row of *nine* categories placing at one end of the row those cards you consider *most characteristic* or *salient* with respect to the subject and at the other end, those cards you believe to be *most uncharacteristic* or *negatively salient* with reference to the subject.

A convenient method of sorting is to first form three stacks of cards—those items deemed characteristic being placed on one side, those items deemed uncharacteristic being placed on the other side, and those cards remaining falling in between. No attention need be paid to the number of cards falling into each of these three groupings

138

The number of cards to be placed in each category are:

Category	No. of Cards	Label of Category
9	5	extremely characteristic or salient
8	8	quite characteristic or salient
7	12	fairly characteristic or salient
6	16	somewhat characteristic or salient
5	18	relatively neutral or unimportant
4	16	somewhat uncharacteristic or negatively salient
3	12	fairly uncharacteristic or negatively salient
2	8	quite uncharacteristic or negatively salient
1	5	extremely uncharacteristic or negatively salient

at this time. When the three piles of cards have been established, they may be further fractionated, this time into their proper proportions.

You will probably feel resentment at the constraints imposed upon you by the Q-deck and the sorting procedure. In justification, it should be noted that specifying the number of cards to be assigned to each category has proven empirically to be a more valuable procedure than the freer situation where the clinician can assign any number of cards to a category. The Q-items themselves represent a good deal of reflection and advice. They have been phrased to keep the distinction between the manifest and the latent. Items referring to pathology *per se* are not present. Pathological characteristics can be expressed by the extremeness of placement of certain of the statements, however, or by a conjunction of two or more of the items.

The intent in constructing this set of items has been to allow it to express any pattern of personality by means of suitable placement of items and the configuration of statements that consequently is built up. If you find any kind of personality that cannot be suitably described by the item set as presently constituted, we would appreciate hearing about these instances in anticipation of the time when the CQ-set will again be revised. If the CQ-set, presently or in the future, is capable of characterizing fairly the kinds of humanity encountered, then it becomes a language instrument of wide applicability in both research and teaching settings.

Appendix C

A COMPARISON OF THE RESULTS PROVIDED
BY DIFFERENT Q-SETS

The question has frequently arisen in discussions of the Q-sort method, To what extent are the findings provided by a given Q-set a unique function of the properties of that deck? The question is an important one, and justly raised, for if Q-findings can be predicted simply on the basis of *a priori* knowledge of the Q-items, the significance of Q-data is restricted greatly (in certain contexts to the vanishing point).

In this appendix we report a comparison of two quite different Q-decks sorted by the same raters with reference to the same social objects. The study is a small one and properly, it requires replication and extension. Nevertheless, however, the results are of some interest.

The study. In connection with a previous study (Block, 1956) four judges had Q-sorted five political figures, employing for their judgments the IPAR 76-item Q-deck devised by assessment psychologists to permit comprehensive characterizations of personality. The 76 items selected attempted to eliminate redundancy and were the result of a good bit of thought and group discussion.

At a second time, after intervals ranging from one week to two months, each sorter again evaluated the same objects using the IPAR Q-set.

Some three to five months after completing the repeat sortings, the four judges still again sorted the social objects, this time employing a different, 60-item Q-set.

The second Q-set was constructed in a fairly unusual way. A part-time secretary at the Institute of Personality Assessment and Research, at the time an English major in the University, was asked to compile a list of 60 adjectives she felt were important and comprehensive for the description of personality. She was allowed 40 minutes for the task. Her selection of adjectives was used without editing or revision of any kind as the second Q-set. The nature of the items included is suggested by listing the first five adjectives.

1. acquisitive
2. adaptable
3. affectionate
4. aggressive
5. ambitious

There are two ways of evaluating the extent of functional equivalence of the two sets. The first is simply to list for a given sorter and a given object the extremely placed items for both Q-sets. An impressionistic appraisal is then possible of the extent to which the same portrayals are being offered, even if in different terms. An illustration of this approach is presented below.

With the IPAR Q-set (initial sort), Rater A employed the following eight items as *most* characteristic of Object V. These represent the first two intervals, consisting of three and five items respectively, of a nine step continuum.

11. Is a conscientious, responsible, dependable person.
32. Highly cathects intellectual activity; values cognitive pursuits.
71. Communicates ideas clearly and effectively.
2. Has high degree of intellectual ability.
3. Is an effective leader.
18. Efficient, capable, able to mobilize resources easily and effectively; not bothered with work inhibitions.
22. Is verbally fluent; conversationally facile.
57. Tends to take stands on moral grounds and issues.

Rater A employed the eight IPAR Q-set items listed below as *least* characteristic of Object V.

6. Is guileful and potentially deceitful.
7. Has a narrow range of interests.
56. Is pedantic and fussy about minor things.
12. Manipulates people as a means to achieving personal ends; opportunistic; sloughs over the meaning and value of the individual.
17. Is rigid; inflexible in thought and action.
20. Lacks social poise and presence; becomes rattled and upset in social situations.

45. Under-controls his impulses; acts with insufficient thinking and deliberation; unable to delay gratification.
66. Emphasizes oral pleasure; self-indulgent.

Using the second Q-set, the six most characteristic and the six least characteristic items are:

Most Characteristic	*Least Characteristic*
11. creative	50. smug
27. intelligent	55. timid
2. adaptable	23. hostile
18. forthright	40. pompous
24. imaginative	51. strait-laced
48. sense of humor	59. willful

It is difficult to estimate the degree of equivalence between these characterizations of a personality. There are a number of intuitively clear agreements between the two listings and no apparent disagreements. But there appear to be a number of personality facets indicated as extremely salient in one Q-set but not manifestly paralleled or so extremely judged in the other set. The non-comparability of the languages used in the separate Q-sets prevents a clear estimation of their equivalence. For this reason, the second method of evaluation is to be favored.

A fundamental test of the functional equivalence of two sets of data is the existence of an isomorphism of the relationships among the variables constituting each data-set. That is, if there exists a strong relationship between subjects A and B in one data-set, there should also exist a strong relationship between these same subjects in the second data-set. An over-all method for characterizing the degree of isomorphism is to simply treat the correlation between subjects as *scores* and correlate all of these scores paired across data-sets. The coefficient resulting from this inter-matrix correlation is thus an index of the functional equivalence or similarity of covariation of the two sets of data.

For each sorter, the matrices based upon the IPAR Q-set (initial sorting), the IPAR Q-set (repeat sorting) and secretary's Q-set were inter-correlated. Each matrix was of order 5 x 5, and consequently an N of only 10 (i.e., 10 separate cells) was involved in the rank-order correlations. These correlations are presented in Table 7.

Table 7

Inter-matrix Correlations of Q-set Data

Rater	Correlation of initial and repeat matrices employing the IPAR Q-set	Correlation of initial matrix based upon the IPAR Q-set and matrix based upon the secretary's Q-set	Correlation of repeat matrix based upon the IPAR Q-set and matrix based upon the secretary's Q-set
A	.75	.82	.96
B	.99	.97	.98
C	.90	.61	.67
D	.60	.74	.76

The inter-matrix correlations of the IPAR Q-set, initial versus repeat sortings, provides a reference frame in terms of which the IPAR Q-set and secretary's Q-set correlations can be interpreted. The correspondence between the matrices of the two different Q-sets is of the same degree as the correspondence between the IPAR Q-set (initial) and the IPAR Q-set (repeat) matrices. Clearly, then, these data suggest that the nature of the covariation among objects when the IPAR Q-set was employed is no different from the nature of the covariation among objects when the secretary's Q-set was used.

Discussion. By no means can the findings of this tiny and circumscribed study be generalized to the far reaches of possible Q-applications. The inter-matrix correlations are based on very small N's (although this introduces no bias in the results) and sampling fortuities might well explain away the result. It would be well to repeat and extend this study in a variety of ways to test this initial finding fairly.

Most particularly, it should be remembered that although the two Q-sets compared were constructed in quite different ways and terms, the universe which each attempted to encompass was the same. Where the defined domains differ (e.g., manifest versus inferred characteristics) it is more likely that Q-set comparisons will not show functional equivalence.

Appendix D

A CQ-SET DESCRIPTION OF THE OPTIMALLY ADJUSTED PERSONALITY, AS VIEWED BY CLINICAL PSYCHOLOGISTS

In establishing a consensually-based description of optimal adjustment and also in deriving the descriptions of male paranoia and female hysteria, in Appendices E and F, nine clinical psychologists were employed.* All held the Ph.D. degree and appreciable clinical experience in a variety of settings. It seems fair to say that as a group this sample is reasonably representative of the views and conceptions held by contemporary clinical psychologists. To the extent that representativeness may be assumed, it follows that the conceptual definitions derived from this group may serve as a criterion against which individual formulations of the concept may be compared.

The average inter-correlation among the nine definitions of optimal adjustment was .78, implying by the Spearman-Brown formula that the realiability of the composite description is .97. Individual clinicians, who on the average are equivalent to those contributing toward the consensual definition, may expect their own formulations of optimal adjustment to correlate about .87 with the composite.

For the reader's immediate convenience, the thirteen CQ-items (categories 9 and 8) deemed *most characteristic* of the optimally adjusted personality and the thirteen items (categories 1 and 2) considered to be *most uncharacteristic* are listed below.

CQ-items considered as positively defining of optimal adjustment:

35. Has warmth; has the capacity for close relationships; compassionate.

2. Is a genuinely dependable and responsible person.

60. Has insight into own motives and behavior.

---

* I am much indebted, for their help in defining these concepts, to Doctors Bernard Apfelbaum, Jeanne Block, Wanda Bronson, Orin G. Dalaba, Curt Hardyck, Shirley Hecht, Mary D. Rauch and Elaine Simpson. The counting reader will be able to infer that I provided the ninth set of conceptual descriptions.

26. Is productive; gets things done.
64. Is socially perceptive of a wide range of interpersonal cues.
70. *Behaves* in an ethically consistent manner; is consistent with own personal standards.
96. Values own independence and autonomy.
77. Appears straightforward, forthright, candid in dealings with others.
83. Able to see to the heart of important problems.
51. Genuinely values intellectual and cognitive matters. (N.B. Ability or achievement are not implied here.)
33. Is calm, relaxed in manner.
17. Behaves in a sympathetic or considerate manner.
 3. Has a wide range of interests. (N.B. Superficiality or depth of interest is irrelevant here.)

CQ-items considered as negatively defining of optimal adjustment:
45. Has a brittle ego-defense system; has a small reserve of integration: would be disorganized and maladaptive when under stress or trauma.
78. Feels cheated and victimized by life; self-pitying.
86. Handles anxiety and conflicts by, in effect, refusing to recognize their presence; repressive or dissociative tendencies.
22. Feels a lack of personal meaning in life.
55. Is self-defeating.
40. Is vulnerable to real or fancied threat, generally fearful.
48. Keeps people at a distance; avoids close interpersonal relationships.
68. Is basically anxious.
37. Is guileful and deceitful, manipulative, opportunistic.
36. Is subtly negativistic; tends to undermine and obstruct or sabotage.
38. Has hostility towards others. (N.B. Basic hostility is intended here; mode of expression is to be indicated by other items).
76. Tends to project his own feelings and motivations onto others.
97. Is emotionally bland; has flattened effect.

The complete description of optimal adjustment is recorded on the next page. Two entries appear for each CQ-item. The first is the average value assigned to the item by the nine judges. The second figure represents the category value of the item, after the set of 100 item means is "re-Q'ed" into the standard CQ-distribution. For hand-calculated estimations of correspondence involving this composite, the latter set of entries is especially useful.

California Q-set Record Sheet

Subject: The Optimally Adjusted Personality   Sorter: _____   9 Psychologists' Consensus   Informational source: _____   The concept, as understood _____   Date: _____

Item	Value	Cat	Item	Value	Cat	Item	Value	Cat	Item	Value	Cat	Item	Value	Cat
1	5.8	6	21	4.7	5	41	4.3	4	61	3.1	3	81	5.0	5
2	8.8	9	22	1.9	1	42	3.1	3	62	5.0	5	82	4.4	5
3	7.1	8	23	3.1	3	43	6.2	6	63	3.8	4	83	7.3	8
4	5.0	5	24	5.6	5	44	6.7	7	64	7.9	9	84	6.9	7
5	6.4	7	25	3.3	3	45	1.0	1	65	3.4	4	85	4.7	5
6	5.0	5	26	8.3	9	46	5.2	5	66	7.0	7	86	1.9	1
7	4.6	5	27	2.9	3	47	3.2	3	67	5.7	5	87	3.8	4
8	6.1	6	28	7.1	7	48	2.3	2	68	2.3	2	88	6.0	6
9	3.3	3	29	6.0	6	49	3.1	3	69	4.2	4	89	4.2	4
10	3.0	3	30	3.6	4	50	4.1	4	70	7.9	8	90	6.4	6
11	6.3	6	31	5.7	5	51	7.2	8	71	6.4	6	91	4.9	5
12	3.1	3	32	6.7	7	52	6.0	6	72	3.8	4	92	6.9	7
13	3.0	3	33	7.2	8	53	3.7	4	73	4.3	4	93	6.3	6
14	4.1	4	34	3.4	4	54	5.4	5	74	5.9	6	94	5.8	6
15	6.6	7	35	8.9	9	55	2.0	1	75	6.2	6	95	4.8	5
16	6.0	6	36	2.4	2	56	6.8	7	76	2.7	2	96	7.7	8
17	7.2	8	37	2.4	2	57	6.7	7	77	7.6	8	97	2.7	2
18	6.2	6	38	2.6	2	58	6.8	7	78	1.4	1	98	6.1	6
19	4.8	5	39	5.4	5	59	3.9	4	79	3.3	3	99	4.1	4
20	5.2	5	40	2.1	2	60	8.4	9	80	6.9	7	100	4.0	4

Specified CQ distribution

Category value	1	2	3	4	5	6	7	8	9
Number of items in category	5	8	12	16	18	16	12	8	5

Formula for correlation between CQ sorts: $r = 1 - \dfrac{\text{sum } d^2}{864}$

N.B. A value of 9 indicates "most characteristic", a value of 1 indicates "least characteristic".

A CQ-SET DESCRIPTION OF THE MALE PARANOID, AS VIEWED BY CLINICAL PSYCHOLOGISTS

The psychologists mentioned in Appendix D provided the nine separate descriptions of male paranoia used to develop the present composite description. The average inter-correlation among the nine definitions was .55, appreciably lower than the average agreement recorded for the descriptions of optimal adjustment. Nevertheless, application of the Spearman-Brown formula indicates that the reliability of the composite is .92, a quite satisfactory figure. Individual clinicians who on the average are equivalent to those contributing toward this consensual definition may expect their own descriptions to correlate about .71 with the composite.

For the reader's immediate convenience, the thirteen CQ-items (categories 9 and 8) deemed *most characteristic* of the male paranoid and the thirteen items (categories 1 and 2) considered to be *most uncharacteristic* are listed below.

CQ-items considered as positively defining of male paranoia:

49. Is basically distrustful of people in general; questions their motivations.
76. Tends to project his own feelings and motivations onto others.
38. Has hostility toward others. (N.B. Basic hostility is intended here; mode of expression is to be indicated by other items).
23. Extrapunitive; tends to transfer or project blame.
48. Keeps people at a distance; avoids close interpersonal relationships.
68. Is basically anxious.
13. Is thin-skinned; sensitive to anything that can be construed as criticism or an interpersonal slight.
41. Is moralistic. (N.B. Regardless of the particular nature of the moral code.)

79. Tends to ruminate and have persistent, preoccupying thoughts.

72. Concerned with own adequacy as a person, either at conscious or unconscious levels. (N.B. A clinical judgment is required here; number 74 reflects subjective satisfaction with self.)

91. Is power oriented; values power in self or others.

24. Prides self on being "objective," rational.

87. Interprets basically simple and clear-cut situations in complicated and particularizing ways.

CQ-items considered as negatively defining of the male paranoid:

60. Has insight into own motives and behavior.

14. *Genuinely* submissive; accepts domination comfortably.

21. Arouses nurturant feelings in others.

35. Has warmth; has the capacity for close relationships; compassionate.

58. Enjoys sensuous experiences (including touch, taste, smell, physical contact).

5. Behaves in a giving way toward others. (N.B. regardless of the motivation involved.)

28. Tends to arouse liking and acceptance in people.

84. Is cheerful. (N.B. Extreme placement toward uncharacteristic end of continuum implies unhappiness or depression.)

33. Is calm, relaxed in manner.

18. Initiates humor.

17. Behaves in a sympathetic or considerate manner.

77. Appears straightforward, forthright, candid in dealings with others.

54. Emphasizes being with others; gregarious.

The complete description of male paranoia is recorded on the next page. Two entries appear for each CQ-item. The first is the average value assigned to the item by the nine judges. The second figure represents the category value of the item, after the set of 100 item means is "re-Q'ed" into the standard CQ-distribution.

California Q-set Record Sheet

9 Psychologists' Consensus

Subject: The Male Paranoid Sorter: _____ Informational source; The concept, as understood _____ Date: _____

1	2	3	4	5	6	7	8	9	10	11	12	13	14	15	16	17	18	19	20
6.3 7	3.1 3	4.2 4	4.9 5	2.8 2	5.3 6	5.6 6	5.7 6	6.4 7	4.1 4	3.8 4	6.6 7	7.2 8	2.0 1	3.7 3	4.9 5	3.0 2	2.9 2	3.6 3	4.4 4

21	22	23	24	25	26	27	28	29	30	31	32	33	34	35	36	37	38	39	40
2.7 1	4.1 4	8.1 9	7.0 8	6.2 6	4.7 5	6.2 6	2.8 2	3.6 3	3.2 3	4.7 5	4.3 4	2.9 2	6.2 6	2.7 1	5.8 6	5.0 5	8.1 9	6.8 7	6.3 7

41	42	43	44	45	46	47	48	49	50	51	52	53	54	55	56	57	58	59	60
7.1 8	4.2 4	3.6 3	6.3 7	6.7 7	6.2 6	3.7 3	8.1 9	8.7 9	4.6 5	5.0 5	5.8 6	3.4 3	3.1 2	5.8 6	3.7 3	4.9 5	2.7 1	5.0 5	1.8 1

61	62	63	64	65	66	67	68	69	70	71	72	73	74	75	76	77	78	79	80
5.2 5	4.9 5	4.4 4	4.4 5	4.0 4	3.8 4	3.7 3	7.4 8	6.6 7	4.4 4	6.2 7	7.0 8	5.7 6	5.4 6	4.1 4	8.3 9	3.1 2	6.8 7	7.0 8	3.3 3

81	82	83	84	85	86	87	88	89	90	91	92	93	94	95	96	97	98	99	100
4.9 5	5.1 5	3.8 4	2.9 2	5.0 5	6.1 6	6.9 8	3.9 4	6.8 7	6.1 6	7.0 8	4.0 4	5.2 5	3.6 3	5.7 6	6.7 7	4.4 4	5.2 5	5.3 5	5.6 6

Specified CQ distribution

Category value	1	2	3	4	5	6	7	8	9
Number of items in category	5	8	12	16	18	16	12	8	5

Formula for correlation between CQ sorts: $r = 1 - \dfrac{\text{sum } d^2}{864}$

N.B. A value of 9 indicates "most characteristic"; a value of 1 indicates "least characteristic".

A CQ-SET DESCRIPTION OF THE FEMALE HYSTERIC, AS VIEWED BY CLINICAL PSYCHOLOGISTS

The psychologists listed in Appendix D provided the nine separate descriptions of the female hysteric used to construct the present consensus definition. The average inter-correlation among the nine formulations was .51, slightly lower than the agreement figure achieved by these clinicians in defining paranoia and substantially lower than the agreement figure registered in defining optimal adjustment. The cumulative import of these nine descriptions is quite substantial however, for the Spearman-Brown estimate of the reliability of the composite is .91. Individual clinicians who on the average are equivalent to those contributing toward this consensus may expect their own descriptions to correlate about .68 with the composite.

For the reader's immediate convenience, the thirteen CQ-items (categories 9 and 8) deemed *most characteristic* of the female hysteric and the thirteen items (categories 1 and 2) considered to be *most uncharacteristic* are listed below.

CQ-items considered as positively defining of the female hysteric:

86. Handles anxiety and conflicts by, in effect, refusing to recognize their presence; repressive or dissociative tendencies.
99. Is self-dramatizing histrionic.
93b. *Behaves* in a feminine style and manner.
63. Judges self and others in conventional terms like "popularity," "the correct thing to do," social pressures, etc.
12. Tends to be self-defensive.
9. Is uncomfortable with uncertainty and complexities.
54. Emphasizes being with others; gregarious.
68. Is basically anxious.
72. Concerned with own adequacy as a person, either at conscious or unconscious levels. (N.B. A clinical judgment is required here; number 74 reflects subjective satisfaction with self.)

10. Anxiety and tension find outlet in bodily symptoms. (N.B. If placed high, implies bodily dysfunction; if placed low, implies absence of autonomic arousal.)
19. Seeks reassurance from others.
59. Is concerned with own body and the adequacy of its physiological functioning.
41. Is moralistic. (N.B. Regardless of the particular nature of the moral code.)

CQ-items considered as negatively defining of the female hysteric:
60. Has insight into own motives and behavior.
83. Able to see to the heart of important problems.
 1. Is critical, skeptical, not easily impressed.
94. Expresses hostile feelings directly.
39. Thinks and associates to ideas in unusual ways; has unconventional thought processes.
79. Tends to ruminate and have persistent, preoccupying thoughts.
64. Is socially perceptive of a wide range of interpersonal cues.
33. Is calm, relaxed in manner.
62. Tends to be rebellious and non-conforming.
16. Is introspective and concerned with self as an object. (N.B. introspectiveness *per se* does not imply insight.)
35. Has warmth; has the capacity for close relationships; compassionate.
77. Appears straightforward, forthright, candid in dealings with others.
90. Is concerned with philosophical problems; e.g., religions, values, the meaning of life, etc.

The complete description of the female hysteric is recorded on the next page. Two entries appear for each CQ-item. The first is the average value assigned to the item by the nine judges. The second figure represents the category value of the item, after the set of 100 item means is "re-Q'ed" into the standard CQ-distribution.

California Q-set Record Sheet

Subject: __The Female Hysteric__   Sorter: _____   9 Psychologists' Consensus   Informational source: __The concept, as understood__   Date: _____

1	2	3	4	5	6	7	8	9	10	11	12	13	14	15	16	17	18	19	20
2.2	3.9	3.7	6.3	4.2	5.2	6.4	4.4	7.3	7.0	4.2	7.6	6.0	4.2	5.3	2.9	4.6	4.8	7.0	5.4
1	3	3	7	4	6	7	4	8	8	4	9	6	4	6	2	4	5	8	6

21	22	23	24	25	26	27	28	29	30	31	32	33	34	35	36	37	38	39	40
4.9	3.9	5.9	4.6	4.8	4.1	4.9	5.0	3.3	5.8	5.6	3.8	2.8	5.0	3.0	6.4	5.4	6.7	2.6	5.8
5	3	6	4	5	3	5	5	3	6	6	3	2	5	2	7	6	7	1	6

41	42	43	44	45	46	47	48	49	50	51	52	53	54	55	56	57	58	59	60
6.8	4.1	6.6	3.1	6.0	4.8	4.4	4.7	4.3	5.9	3.6	4.3	4.3	7.2	5.2	5.1	4.3	4.1	6.9	1.0
8	4	7	3	6	5	4	5	4	6	3	4	4	8	6	5	4	4	8	1

61	62	63	64	65	66	67	68	69	70	71	72	73	74	75	76	77	78	79	80
5.6	2.8	7.6	2.7	4.3	4.7	5.8	7.2	5.2	3.3	5.0	7.1	6.4	6.8	3.7	5.8	3.1	5.1	2.6	6.6
6	2	9	2	4	5	6	8	6	3	5	8	7	7	3	6	2	5	2	7

81	82	83	84	85	86	87	88	89	90	91	92	93	94	95	96	97	98	99	100
5.2	6.6	2.2	6.2	6.7	9.0	3.8	4.8	6.6	3.1	5.0	5.0	7.7	2.3	5.1	4.1	4.9	4.2	8.2	4.4
5	7	1	7	7	9	3	5	7	2	5	5	9	1	5	3	5	4	9	4

Specified CQ distribution

Category value	1	2	3	4	5	6	7	8	9
Number of items in category	5	8	12	16	18	16	12	8	5

Formula for correlation between CQ sorts: $r = 1 - \dfrac{\text{sum } d^2}{864}$

N.B. A value of 9 indicates "most characteristic"; a value of 1 indicates "least characteristic".

Appendix G

TABLE FOR CONVERTING SUM OF SQUARED DISCREPANCIES INTO *R*, WHERE THE CQ-DISTRIBUTION IS EMPLOYED

Sum d_{iD}^2	r	Sum d_{iD}^2	r	Sum d_{iD}^2	r	Sum d_{iD}^2	r
0- 4	1.00	428-436	.50	860-868	.00	1292-1300	— .50
5- 12	.99	437-444	.49	869-876	—.01	1301-1308	— .51
13- 21	.98	445-453	.48	877-885	—.02	1309-1317	— .52
22- 30	.97	454-462	.47	886-894	—.03	1318-1326	— .53
31- 38	.96	463-470	.46	895-902	—.04	1327-1334	— .54
39- 47	.95	471-479	.45	903-911	—.05	1335-1343	— .55
48- 56	.94	480-488	.44	912-920	—.06	1344-1352	— .56
57- 64	.93	489-496	.43	921-928	—.07	1353-1360	— .57
65- 73	.92	497-505	.42	929-937	—.08	1361-1369	— .58
74- 82	.91	506-514	.41	938-946	—.09	1370-1378	— .59
83- 90	.90	515-522	.40	947-954	—.10	1379-1386	— .60
91- 99	.89	523-531	.39	955-963	—.11	1387-1395	— .61
100-108	.88	532-539	.38	964-971	—.12	1396-1403	— .62
109-116	.87	540-548	.37	972-980	—.13	1404-1412	— .63
117-125	.86	549-557	.36	981-989	—.14	1413-1421	— .64
126-133	.85	558-565	.35	990-997	—.15	1422-1429	— .65
134-142	.84	566-574	.34	998-1006	—.16	1430-1438	— .66
143-151	.83	575-583	.33	1007-1015	—.17	1439-1447	— .67
152-159	.82	584-591	.32	1016-1023	—.18	1448-1455	— .68
160-168	.81	592-600	.31	1024-1032	—.19	1456-1464	— .69
169-177	.80	601-609	.30	1033-1041	—.20	1465-1473	— .70
178-185	.79	610-617	.29	1042-1049	—.21	1474-1481	— .71
186-194	.78	618-626	.28	1050-1058	—.22	1482-1490	— .72
195-203	.77	627-635	.27	1059-1067	—.23	1491-1499	— .73
204-211	.76	636-643	.26	1068-1075	—.24	1500-1507	— .74
212-220	.75	644-652	.25	1076-1084	—.25	1508-1516	— .75
221-228	.74	653-660	.24	1085-1092	—.26	1517-1524	— .76
229-237	.73	661-669	.23	1093-1101	—.27	1525-1533	— .77
238-246	.72	670-678	.22	1102-1110	—.28	1534-1542	— .78
247-254	.71	679-686	.21	1111-1118	—.29	1543-1550	— .79
255-263	.70	687-695	.20	1119-1127	—.30	1551-1559	— .80
264-272	.69	696-704	.19	1128-1136	—.31	1560-1568	— .81
273-280	.68	705-712	.18	1137-1144	—.32	1569-1576	— .82
281-289	.67	713-721	.17	1145-1153	—.33	1577-1585	— .83
290-298	.66	722-730	.16	1154-1162	—.34	1586-1594	— .84
299-306	.65	731-738	.15	1163-1170	—.35	1595-1603	— .85
307-315	.64	739-747	.14	1171-1179	—.36	1603-1611	— .86
316-323	.63	748-755	.13	1180-1187	—.37	1612-1619	— .87
324-332	.62	756-764	.12	1188-1196	—.38	1620-1628	— .88
333-341	.61	765-773	.11	1197-1205	—.39	1629-1637	— .89
342-349	.60	774-781	.10	1206-1214	—.40	1638-1645	— .90
350-358	.59	782-790	.09	1215-1222	—.41	1646-1654	— .91
359-367	.58	791-799	.08	1223-1231	—.42	1655-1663	— .92
368-375	.57	800-807	.07	1232-1239	—.43	1664-1671	— .93
376-384	.56	808-816	.06	1240-1248	—.44	1672-1680	— .94
385-393	.55	817-825	.05	1249-1257	—.45	1681-1689	— .95
394-401	.54	826-833	.04	1258-1265	—.46	1690-1697	— .96
402-410	.53	834-842	.03	1266-1274	—.47	1698-1706	— .97
411-419	.52	843-851	.02	1275-1283	—.48	1707-1715	— .98
420-427	.51	852-859	.01	1284-1291	—.49	1716-1723	— .99
						1724-1732	—1.00

AN ADJECTIVE Q-SET FOR USE BY NON-PROFESSIONAL SORTERS (FORM III) SPECIFIED 7-POINT DISTRIBUTION (N—70): 10 ADJECTIVES IN EACH CATEGORY

$$r = 1 - \frac{\text{Sum } d_{ip}^2}{560}$$

1. absent-minded
2. affected
3. ambitious
4. assertive, dominant
5. bossy
6. calm
7. cautious
8. competitive
9. confident
10. considerate
11. cooperative
12. cruel, mean
13. defensive
14. dependent
15. disorderly
16. dissatisfied
17. dramatic
18. dull
19. easily embarrassed
20. easily hurt
21. energetic
22. fair-minded, objective
23. feminine
24. frank
25. friendly
26. guileful
27. helpless
28. hostile
29. idealistic
30. imaginative
31. impulsive
32. intelligent
33. versatile
34. introspective
35. jealous
36. lazy
37. likable
38. persevering
39. personally charming
40. reasonable
41. rebellious
42. resentful
43. reserved, dignified
44. restless
45. sarcastic
46. poised
47. self-controlled
48. self-indulgent
49. selfish
50. self-pitying
51. sense of humor
52. sentimental
53. shrewd, clever
54. sincere
55. sophisticated
56. stubborn
57. suspicious
58. sympathetic
59. timid, submissive
60. touchy, irritable
61. tactless
62. unconventional
63. undecided, confused
64. unhappy
65. uninterested, indifferent
66. unworthy, inadequate
67. warm
68. withdrawn, introverted
69. worried and anxious
70. wise

You have been asked to describe yourself as you honestly see yourself. You are to use the adjectives listed on the next page. Please read the instructions through several times since it is important that the procedure be followed in all its detail.

Look through the list of adjectives and notice that a good many of them are descriptive of you, to a greater or lesser degree. Other of the adjectives are quite undescriptive of you and are even the opposite of the way you see yourself. Your task is to indicate the various *degrees* with which each adjective describes you.

As a first step, look through the list and then pick out the *ten* adjectives or phrases you feel are most characteristic or descriptive of you. Put the number 7 in front of these words. Now, look through the list again and pick out the *ten* words which you feel are quite characteristic of you (excluding from consideration those words you have already given the number 7 to). Write the number 6 in front of these words. Now of those words that remain, pick out the *ten* adjectives that you feel are fairly descriptive of you and place the number 5 in front of them.

Now work from the opposite end toward the middle. Of those words not yet numbered, pick out the *ten* adjectives that are most uncharacteristic of you and give them the number *1*. Pick out the *ten* adjectives that you feel are quite uncharacteristic of you and give them the number *2*. Now choose the *ten* adjectives fairly uncharacteristic of you and give them the number *3*.

As a check, count the words that still have no numbers. If the total is *ten* then you have followed the procedure properly. If the total is different, then a mistake has been made somewhere and you had better check to see if you have ten words numbered 7, ten 6's, ten 5's, ten 3's, ten 2's, ten 1's.

When you have checked to see if you are correct, place the number 4 in front of the ten words remaining without numbers and your task is finished.

A few warning words. You may have difficulty in placing the required number of adjectives into each of the categories. For example, where ten words are required for a category, you may find that you have too many or too few. In either event, finish with the required number of words, either by eliminating those that can most sensibly be moved out or by moving in those words that are most relevant. You may feel that some of your word placements are forced. Your task is admittedly an awkward one but try and work through it anyway. There is a research method in our madness.

In closing we should like to emphasize again that the worth of this research is completely dependent upon how well and conscientiously the various people participating in it carry through their tasks. Numbering the adjectives as described above is perhaps tedious. When honestly done, the results can be quite self-revealing. By the method of coding being used, no one can know just how you honestly evaluate yourself. We would request therefore that if for some reason you feel that you cannot or prefer not to carry through with this task in a meaningful and honest manner, mail in the material with a simple note to this effect. As you can readily see, an analysis of adjectives which have been jokingly numbered or very cautiously responded to would prove to be worthless. Thank you for your cooperation.

INDEX

TEXAS A&M UNIVERSITY - TEXARKANA